STRESS, ANXIETY, AND INSOMNIA

WHAT THE DRUG COMPANIES WON'T TELL YOU AND YOUR DOCTOR DOESN'T KNOW

THE NATURAL SOLUTIONS THAT CAN CHANGE YOUR LIFE

MICHAEL T. MURRAY, N.D.

STRESS, ANXIETY, AND INSOMNIA
WHAT THE DRUG COMPANIES WON'T TELL YOU AND YOUR DOCTOR DOESN'T KNOW

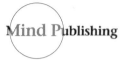

Our focus is education

COPYRIGHT © 2012 MICHAEL T. MURRAY, N.D.

FOR INFORMATION CONTACT

Mind Publishing Inc.
PO Box 57559,
1031 Brunette Avenue
Coquitlam, BC Canada V3K 1E0
Tel: 604-777-4330 Toll free: 1-877-477-4904
Fax: 1-866-367-5508
Email: info@mindpublishing.com
www.mindpublishing.com

ISBN: 978-1-927017-07-4
Printed in Canada

Design: FWH Creative
Editor: Shelagh Jamieson

TABLE OF CONTENTS

Acknowledgments I

Foreword III

Preface V

CHAPTER 1 – What is Stress? 1

Recognizing Stress 2

Understanding Stress 2

The General Adaptation Syndrome 2

Stress: A Healthy View 4

Can Stress be Measured? 5

Effective Stress Management 6

CHAPTER 2 – Develop Positive Coping Strategies 9

Chemical Dependencies 10

Seven Steps to a Stress-Busting Attitude 12

Calming the Mind and Body 18

Learning How to Breathe 20

Progressive Relaxation 21

CHAPTER 3 – Get a Good Night's Sleep 23

Sleep Deprivation in the United States 24

The Problem with Sleeping Pills 24

Improving Sleep Quality Naturally 28

Melatonin 30

5-HTP 31

L-theanine 31

Valerian 32

CHAPTER 4 – Stabilize Blood Sugar Levels 35

Understanding Blood Sugar Control 35

What Does All This Biochemistry Have to Do with Stress? 37

The Negative Effects of Excess Cortisol 38

Stabilizing Blood Sugar Levels is a Key to Stress Management _____ 40

PGX® is the Key _____ 42

Eat to Support Blood Sugar Control _____ 44

CHAPTER 5 – Nourish Your Body and Brain _____ 47

Key Dietary Recommendations _____ 48

Key Nutrients to Protect Against Stress _____ 53

CHAPTER 6 – Manage Your Life _____ 63

The Importance of Time Management _____ 64

Stress and Relationships _____ 65

Develop Health Habits _____ 66

The Anti-Stress Benefits of Regular Exercise _____ 67

CHAPTER 7 – Use Natural Products _____ 73

Serotonin _____ 74

Antidepressant drugs _____ 75

Alternatives to SSRIs _____ 77

5-HTP _____ 78

SAMe _____ 80

Nutritional Products for Stress and Anxiety _____ 81

L-theanine _____ 83

PharmaGABA _____ 83

Key Botanical Medicines for Stress _____ 85

Ginseng _____ 86

Rhodiola _____ 87

Ashwagandha _____ 88

Lavender _____ 89

CONCLUSIONS _____ 93

APPENDICES _____ 97

Appendix A – The Stress Scale _____ 97

Appendix B – Seligman's Attributional Style Questionnaire _____ 99

Appendix C – Frequently Asked Questions on PGX _____ 109

Appendix D – Glycemic Index, Carbohydrate Content, and Glycemic Load of Selected Foods 117

Appendix E – Optimal Health Food Pyramid _____ 125

REFERENCES _____ 133

ACKNOWLEDGMENTS

To my wife, Gina, for being the answer to so many of my dreams.

To my children, Lexi, Zach, and Addison, for being so incredibly magnificent and for teaching me so much about life.

To Roland Gahler and everyone at Natural Factors for their tremendous friendship and support over the years.

And finally, I am eternally grateful to all the researchers, physicians, and scientists who over the years have strived to better understand the use of natural medicines.

FOREWORD

We live in stressful times. With so much uncertainty in our world and, increasingly, in most of our lives, we all need to understand the dramatic impact of stress on our well-being and on the well-being of those around us. The difference between a life lived to its fullest, filled with anticipation and joy, and a miserable life governed by fears and bitterness, can be directly related to our ability to reduce and manage our stress. We cannot always control the events in our lives and we certainly cannot avoid stressful events altogether. But we can gain awareness of where stress comes from and we can learn how to respond differently to adversity when it inevitably calls.

Learning to manage stress is a skill set that can be acquired through knowledge and practice. Stress management begins by recognizing what stress is and what causes it. In many cases we bring stress on ourselves and we need to learn and practice different behaviors to avoid unnecessary stress. We also need to learn how to respond differently to stressful circumstances. Responding to stressful events more positively usually involves changes in lifestyle, thinking patterns, and our physiological response to stress. When we truly learn to manage our stress, it becomes the spice of life and a catalyst for self-improvement rather than a cause of burnout and despair.

Michael Murray presents a fresh and compelling insight into the many-faceted causes of unhealthy stress, and he lays out a holistic plan to harness the positive power of stress to make it an important ally in personal growth and the achievement of success. As a true clinician, Dr. Murray helps us deal with many of the underlying reasons behind our unhealthy responses to stress, rather than just covering up the symptoms. He then skillfully leads us through practical steps to bring about a transformation in the way that stress impacts our daily life. For anyone whose life is overshadowed by the dark clouds and strong winds of stress, this book is a travel guide that can lead you to places of serenity and sunshine.

MICHAEL R. LYON, M.D.

Adjunct Professor
University of British Columbia
Food, Nutrition, and Health Program

Medical and Research Director
Canadian Centre for Functional Medicine

PREFACE

Stress, anxiety, and insomnia are common to many North Americans. Unfortunately, when most people go to a medical doctor for relief of symptoms of stress, anxiety, or insomnia they are usually prescribed drugs like Xanax, Lunesta, Ambien, or Valium or an antidepressant drug like Prozac, Zoloft, or Paxil. The drug approach is much like a biochemical band-aid that covers up the symptoms, but does not address the underlying cause and in many cases leads to even more problems. It is much more rational to utilize a natural approach that provides better solutions to stress, anxiety, depression, and insomnia.

Very rarely are underlying factors or non-drug measures discussed in a typical office visit with a doctor. Natural measures are not discussed because most doctors have not been adequately educated on the role that diet, lifestyle, and attitude can play in determining an individual's response to stress. And, most doctors know very little about the use of dietary supplements or herbal medicines. So their only tools are drugs, and the drug companies spend huge amounts of money each year convincing doctors they are doing the right thing by emphasizing drug treatment. Unfortunately, this focus on drug therapy is at the expense of non-drug therapies such as psychotherapy, social approaches, and nutritional, herbal, or other alternative therapies.

It is not just the physicians who are at fault here. Patients also feed into the problem. Many patients would much rather solve their problem by taking a pill than by taking personal responsibility for their own health and lifestyle. Obviously, by reading this book you are taking charge of your health and looking for natural ways to improve your life. By doing so, your reward will not only be a healthier life, but also one filled with higher levels of energy, joy, vitality, and a tremendous passion for living.

That said, this book must not be used in place of a physician or qualified health care practitioner. Ideally it is designed for use in conjunction with the services provided by physicians practicing natural medicine. Readers are strongly urged to develop a good relationship with a physician knowledgeable in the art and science of natural and preventive medicine, such as a naturopathic physician. In all cases involving a physical or medical complaint, ailment or therapy, please consult a physician. Proper medical care and advice can significantly improve the quality and duration of your life.

Although this book discusses numerous natural approaches to various health conditions, it is not intended as a substitute for appropriate medical care. Please keep the following in mind as you read:

- **Do not self-diagnose.** If you have concerns about any subject discussed in this book, please consult a physician, preferably a naturopathic doctor (N.D.) or nutritionally oriented medical doctor (M.D.), or a doctor of osteopathy (D.O.), chiropractor (D.C.), or other natural health care specialist.

- **Make your physician aware** of all the nutritional supplements or herbal products you are currently taking to avoid any negative interactions with any drugs you are taking.

- **If you are currently taking a prescription medication**, you absolutely must work with your doctor before discontinuing any drug or altering any drug regimen.

- **Most health conditions require a multi-factorial solution:** medical, nutritional, and lifestyle changes. Do not rely solely on a single area of focus. You can't just take pills and not change your diet, or do the diet and the pills but ignore the lifestyle issues. Any truly effective approach to health must be integrated.

With the above in mind, remember that the information in this book is to be applied, not simply read. Commit yourself to following the guidelines of natural healthcare as detailed in this book and I believe that you will be rewarded immensely.

Michael T. Murray, N.D.
March 2012

CHAPTER 1

WHAT IS STRESS?

All of us know stress. In fact, most of us have accepted the fact that everyday stress is part of modern living. Job pressures; family arguments; financial pressures; and running late are just a few of the "stressors" most of us are faced with on a daily basis. Although we most often think one of these types of stressors are what cause us to feel "stressed out," technically speaking a stressor may be almost any disturbance – heat or cold, environmental toxins, toxins produced by microorganisms, physical trauma, a strong emotional reaction – that can trigger a number of biological changes to produce what is commonly known as the "stress response."

Fortunately for us, control mechanisms in the body are geared toward counteracting the everyday stresses of life. Most often the stress response is so mild it goes entirely unnoticed. However, if stress is extreme, unusual, or long lasting, these control mechanisms can be overwhelming and quite harmful. In these situations especially it is critical to utilize natural approaches to reduce stress and its effects.

RECOGNIZING STRESS

Have you ever been suddenly frightened? That is the extreme end of the stress response. What you were feeling was adrenaline surging through your body. Adrenaline is released from your adrenal glands, a pair of glands that lie on top of each kidney. Adrenaline was designed to give the body that extra energy boost to escape from danger. Unfortunately, it can also make us feel stressed, anxious, and nervous.

In modern life many people experience stress, but may not be able to tell you exactly what it is that is causing them to feel stressed out. What these people may be noticing are the side effects of stress, such as insomnia, depression, fatigue, headache, upset stomach, digestive disturbances, and irritability.

UNDERSTANDING STRESS

Before discussing methods and tools for dealing effectively with stress, it is important to understand the stress response. Ultimately, the success of any stress management program is dependent on its ability to improve an individual's immediate and long-term response to stress.

The stress response is actually part of a larger response known as the "general adaptation syndrome." To fully understand how to combat stress, it is important that we take a closer look at the general adaptation syndrome. The general adaptation syndrome is broken down into three phases: alarm, resistance, and exhaustion. These phases are largely controlled and regulated by the adrenal glands and our nervous system.

THE GENERAL ADAPTATION SYNDROME

The initial response to stress is the alarm reaction that is often referred to as the "fight or flight response." The fight or flight response is triggered by reactions in the brain which ultimately cause the pituitary gland (the master gland of the entire hormonal system of the body, which is located at the center of the base of the brain) to release a hormone called adrenocorticotropic hormone (ACTH) which causes the adrenals to secrete adrenaline and other stress-related hormones, like cortisol.

The fight or flight response is designed to counteract danger by mobilizing the body's resources for immediate physical activity. As a result, the heart rate and force of contraction of the heart increases to provide blood to the areas that may need to response to the stressful situation. Blood is shunted away from the skin and internal organs, except the heart and lung, while at the same time the amount of blood supplying needed oxygen and glucose to the muscles and brain is increased. The rate of breathing increases to supply necessary oxygen to the heart, brain, and exercising muscle. Sweat production increases to eliminate toxic compounds produced by the body and to lower body temperature. Production of digestive secretions is severely reduced since digestive activity is not critical for counteracting stress. And, blood sugar levels are increased dramatically as the liver dumps stored glucose into the bloodstream to provide a quick and easy source of energy.

While the alarm phase is usually short-lived, the next phase – the resistance reaction – allows the body to continue fighting a stressor long after the effects of the fight or flight response have worn off. Other hormones, such as cortisol and other corticosteroids secreted by the adrenal cortex, are largely responsible for the resistance reaction. For example, these hormones stimulate the conversion of protein to energy, so that the body has a large supply of energy long after glucose stores are depleted, as well as promote the retention of sodium to keep blood pressure elevated.

In addition to providing the necessary energy and circulatory changes required to deal effectively with stress, the resistance reaction provides those changes required for meeting an emotional crisis, performing a strenuous task, and fighting infection. However, while the effects of adrenal hormones are quite necessary when the body is faced with danger, prolonging the resistance reaction or continued stress increase the risk of significant disease (including diabetes, high blood pressure, and cancer) and results in the final stage of the general adaptation syndrome: exhaustion.

Prolonged stress places a tremendous load on many organ systems, especially the heart, blood vessels, adrenals, and immune system. Exhaustion may manifest by a total collapse of a body function or a collapse of specific organs.

Table 1.1 – Conditions Strongly Linked to Stress

Angina	Diabetes (adult onset – type 2)	Premenstrual tension syndrome
Asthma	Headaches	Rheumatoid arthritis
Autoimmune disease	Hypertension	Ulcerative colitis
Cancer	Immune suppression	Ulcers
Cardiovascular disease	Irritable bowel syndrome	
Common cold	Menstrual irregularities	
Depression		

STRESS: A HEALTHY VIEW

The "godfather" of modern stress research was Hans Selye, M.D. Having spent most of his life studying stress, this brilliant man probably had the best perspective on the role of stress in our lives. According to Dr. Selye, stress in its self should not be viewed as a negative factor. It is not the stressor that determines the response; instead it is the individual's internal reaction that triggers the response. This internal reaction is highly individualized. What one person may experience as stress, the next person may view entirely differently. Dr. Selye perhaps summarized his view best in this passage from his book *The Stress of Life* (McGraw Hill, New York, NY, 1978):

No one can live without experiencing some degree of stress all the time. You may think that only serious disease or intensive physical or mental injury can cause stress. This is false. Crossing a busy intersection, exposure to a draft, or even sheer joy are enough to activate the body's stress mechanisms to some extent. Stress is not even necessarily bad for you; it is also the spice of life, for any emotion, any activity, causes stress. But, of course, your system must be prepared to take it. The same stress which makes one person sick can be an invigorating experience for another.

The key statement Selye made is "your system must be prepared to take it." It is my goal to help prepare and bolster your stress-fighting system.

CAN STRESS BE MEASURED?

One useful tool to assess the role that stress may play in a person's life is the "social readjustment rating scale" developed by Holmes and Rahe.[1] The scale was originally designed to predict the risk of a serious disease due to stress. Various life-changing events are numerically rated according to their potential to cause disease. To see where you stand on the stress scale, see Appendix A on page 97. You will notice that even events commonly viewed as positive, such as an outstanding personal achievement, carry stress.

Many naturopathic physicians assess stress based on salivary levels of the stress hormone cortisol. Salivary cortisol levels are reproducible, comparable to plasma levels, and easy to assess.[2, 3] Salivary cortisol levels generally show a sharp rise upon awakening and during the first hour after waking up. Generally, an initially overactive acute stress response results in elevated cortisol levels, while more chronic stress, insomnia, or depression may blunt this effect.[4, 5]

Another popular test used in combination with salivary cortisol level testing is measuring DHEA levels. The classic pattern associated with chronic stress is elevated cortisol combined with reduced DHEA, indicating a shift toward stress hormone production and away from sex hormone production. This pattern is often associated with anxiety and depression. Adrenal exhaustion is characterized by low cortisol and low DHEA. Adrenal exhaustion is a common side effect of continual high stress. It is also seen with the use of steroid drugs, like prednisone, in the treatment of allergic or inflammatory diseases.

WHAT IS THE DIFFERENCE BETWEEN STRESS AND ANXIETY?

When we experience stress, it is often accompanied by feelings of anxiety. Technically, anxiety is defined as "an unpleasant emotional state ranging from mild unease to intense fear." Anxiety differs from fear, in that while fear is a rational response to a real danger, anxiety usually lacks a clear or realistic cause. Though some anxiety is normal and, in fact, healthy, higher levels of anxiety are not only uncomfortable, but are linked to all of the issues with long-term stress.

Anxiety is often accompanied by a variety of symptoms. The most common symptoms relate to the chest, such as heart palpitations (awareness of a more forceful or faster heart beat), throbbing or stabbing pains, a feeling of tightness and inability to take in enough air, and a tendency to sigh or hyperventilate. Tension in the muscles of the back and neck often leads to headaches, back pains, and muscle spasms. Other symptoms can include excessive sweating, dryness of the mouth, dizziness, digestive disturbances, and the constant need to urinate or have a bowel movement.

Severe anxiety will often produce what are known as "panic attacks" – intense feelings of fear. Panic attacks may occur independent of anxiety, but are most often associated with generalized anxiety or agoraphobia. Agoraphobia is defined as an intense fear of being in wide-open spaces, crowds, or uncomfortable social situations. As a result, most people with agoraphobia become housebound. How common are panic attacks? Very. It is estimated that about 15% of the United States population experience a panic attack in their lifetime, and 3% report regular panic attacks.

EFFECTIVE STRESS MANAGEMENT

In order to deal with stress effectively it is critical that an individual concentrate on five equally important areas. Lack of attention to any of these key areas will ultimately lead to a breakdown in the system, much as your car requires essential components like tires, a battery, gas, a steering wheel, an engine, and a transmission. Each one of these facets of stress management is very important; as they weave together a cohesive fabric that supports us in dealing with the challenges of life. Undoubtedly, you have heard the saying that a chain is only as strong as its weakest link – well that is certainly true. So, in our stress management program we have to work to make sure that all of the links are strong. Here are the five key areas of focus in developing an effective stress management program:

1. Develop positive coping strategies.
2. Get a good night's sleep.
3. Stabilize blood sugar levels.
4. Nourish your body and brain.
5. Manage your life.

The following chapters detail the specific methods to support these five key areas. Remember, each area is as critical as the next. That said, the list above is somewhat in order of importance. In addition to these areas of focus, sometimes specific natural products can be used to help dampen the stress response and/or support the adrenal glands.

CHAPTER 2

DEVELOP POSITIVE COPING STRATEGIES

Whether you are currently aware of it or not, you have a pattern for coping with stress. Unfortunately, most people have found patterns and methods that ultimately do not support good health. If you are to be truly successful in coping with stress, negative coping patterns must be identified and replaced with the positive ways of coping described in this book. Try to identify below any negative or destructive coping patterns you may have developed:

- Dependence on chemicals
    - Drugs, legal and illicit
    - Alcohol
    - Tobacco
- Overeating

- Too much television
- Emotional outbursts
- Feelings of helplessness
- Overspending
- Excessive behavior

CHEMICAL DEPENDENCIES

The United States appears to be a nation of addicts. The level of addiction ranges from the responsible person who "can't get started in the morning" without a cup of coffee to the strung out crack addict. Check out these sobering statistics.

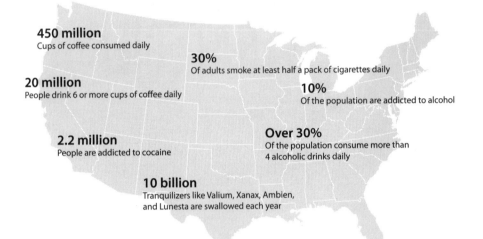

450 million
Cups of coffee consumed daily

30%
Of adults smoke at least half a pack of cigarettes daily

20 million
People drink 6 or more cups of coffee daily

10%
Of the population are addicted to alcohol

2.2 million
People are addicted to cocaine

Over 30%
Of the population consume more than 4 alcoholic drinks daily

10 billion
Tranquilizers like Valium, Xanax, Ambien, and Lunesta are swallowed each year

Often people claim that they smoke, drink alcohol, or take drugs because it calms them. In reality, these substances actually complicate matters. The relaxation or chemical high from these drugs is short-lived and ultimately lead to adding even more stress to the system. Individuals suffering from stress, anxiety, depression, insomnia, or other psychological conditions must absolutely stop drinking coffee and other sources of caffeine, and alcohol. They also need to quit smoking and using recreational drugs. In short, these people must choose health.

THE NEED TO GET HIGH

There appears to be an inherent need for humans to get high. Does this need to be the chemical high that most Americans seek? No. Think back to some fantastic moments in your life. Most of us have experienced an extreme natural high at least once in our lives. What was the moment in your life that seemed almost magical? Was it the first time your wife or lover said they loved you? How about the birth of your first child? Or, how about when you accomplished one of your dreams? Didn't these moments seem almost unreal? Did you feel as if you were naturally high?

All the drugs that act on the brain do so by mimicking or enhancing the activity of natural compounds already present in the brain. Within you lie all the chemicals required for every emotion you can possibly experience. The key is not to take drugs to try to duplicate these feelings, but rather to learn how to create the feelings inside of you so that you can conjure them up whenever you want. Your mind is such a powerful tool in determining how you feel. You can use your mind to create powerful positive emotions that can give you a natural high that can help you cope with stress.

Here is how you can do it. First recreate a powerful positive experience in your life. Do your best to relive those feelings to the fullest. Turn up the dial of intensity as high as you possibly can. Put this book down and do it now.

How do you feel now? It is within you to experience more of the feelings that you really want to have in life. It's easy for us to be moved by incredible feelings of love, appreciation, and energy when we recall powerful positive events in our lives. In particular, I believe that we are wired to experience and express gratitude in our lives. Recalling positive feelings and moments on a regular basis conditions your mind to continue to experience these emotions, which will allow you to be in a more resourceful state of mind when dealing with the stress of life.

All of this may sound a bit funny to you, but believe me it does work. In an effort to provide some guidance in helping you develop a mental attitude that can help deal with stress I offer seven key steps below.

SEVEN STEPS TO A STRESS-BUSTING ATTITUDE

STEP 1 - BECOME AN OPTIMIST

The first step in developing a positive mental attitude is to become an optimist rather than a pessimist. Fortunately, we are, by nature, optimists. Optimism is a vital component of good health and an ally in the healing process. Focus on the positives even in challenging situations. What distinguishes an optimist from a pessimist is the way in which they explain both good and bad events. Dr. Martin Seligman developed a simple test to determine your level of optimism that I am providing as Appendix B on page 99.

STEP 2 - BECOME AWARE OF SELF-TALK

We all talk to ourselves. There is a constant dialogue taking place in our heads. Our self-talk makes an impression on our subconscious mind. In order to develop or maintain a positive mental attitude you must guard against negative self-talk. Become aware of your self-talk and then consciously work to imprint positive self-talk on the subconscious mind. Two powerful tools for creating positive self-talk are questions and affirmations, Steps 3 and 4.

STEP 3 - ASK BETTER QUESTIONS

One of the most powerful tools that I have found useful in improving the quality of self-talk and hence the quality of life, is a series of questions originally given to me by Anthony Robbins, author of the bestsellers *Unlimited Power* and *Awaken the Giant Within*. According to Tony, the quality of your life is equal to the quality of the questions you habitually ask yourself. Tony's assumption is based on his belief that whatever question you ask your brain – you will get an answer.

Let's look at the following example: An individual is met with a particular challenge or problem. He or she can ask a number of questions when in this situation. Questions many people may ask in this circumstance include: "Why does this always happen to me?" Or, "Why am I always so stupid?" Do they get answers to these questions? Do the answers build self-esteem? Does the problem keep reappearing? What would be a higher quality question? How about, "This is a very interesting situation, what do I need to learn from this situation so that it never happens again?" Or, how about "What can I do to make this situation better?"

In another example, let's look at an individual who suffers from depression. What are some questions they might be asking themselves that may not be helping their situation? How about – "Why am I *always* so depressed?" "Why do things *always* seem to go wrong for me?" "Why am I so unhappy?"

What are some better questions they may want to ask themselves? How about – "What do I need to do to gain more enjoyment and happiness in my life?" "What do I need to commit to doing in order to have more happiness and energy in my life?" After they have answered these questions, they should ask themselves this one – "If I had happiness and high energy levels right now, what would it feel like?" – You will be amazed at how powerful questions can be in your life.

When the mind is searching for answers to these questions, it is reprogramming your subconscious into believing you have an abundance of energy. Unless there is a physiological reason for the chronic fatigue, such as anemia, chronic fatigue syndrome, or some serious disease, it won't take long before your subconscious believes.

Regardless of the situation, asking better questions is bound to improve your attitude. If you want to have a better life, simply ask better questions. It sounds simple, because it is. If you want more energy, excitement, and/or happiness in your life, simply ask yourself the following questions on a consistent basis.

1. What am I most happy about in my life right now?
    Why does that make me happy? How does that make me feel?

2. What am I most excited about in my life right now?
    Why does that make me excited? How does that make me feel?

3. What am I most grateful about in my life right now?
    Why does that make me grateful? How does that make me feel?

4. What am I enjoying most about my life right now?
    What about that do I enjoy? How does that make me feel?

5. What am I committed to in my life right now?
    Why am I committed to that? How does that make me feel?

6. Who do I love?
    Who loves me? How does that make me feel?

7. What must I do today to achieve my long-term goal?
    Why is it important for me to achieve my long-term goal? How
    does it make me feel to know that I am making steps to achieve
    my long-term goal?

STEP 4 – EMPLOY POSITIVE AFFIRMATIONS

An affirmation is a statement with some emotional intensity behind it. Positive affirmations can make imprints on the subconscious mind to create a healthy, positive self image. In addition, affirmations can actually fuel the changes you desire. You may want to have the following affirmations in plain sight to recite them over the course of the day:

- I am blessed with an abundance of energy!

- Love, joy, and happiness flow through me with every heartbeat.

- I am thankful to God for all of my good fortune!

- YES I CAN!

Here are some very simple guidelines for creating your own affirmations. Have fun with it! Positive affirmations can make you feel really good if you follow these guidelines.

- Always phrase an affirmation in the present tense. Imagine that it has already come to pass.

- Always phrase the affirmation as a positive statement. Do not use the words not or never.

- Do your best to totally associate with the positive feelings that are generated by the affirmation.

- Keep the affirmation short and simple, but full of feeling. Be creative.

- Imagine yourself really experiencing what you are affirming.

- Make the affirmation personal to you and full of meaning.

Using the above guidelines and examples, write down five affirmations that apply to you. State these affirmations aloud while you are taking your shower or driving, or when you are praying.

STEP 5 – SET POSITIVE GOALS

Learning to set goals is another powerful method for building a positive attitude and raising self-esteem. Goals can be used to create a "success cycle." Achieving goals helps you feel better about yourself, and the better you feel about yourself, the more likely you will achieve your goals. Here are some guidelines to use when setting goals:

STATE THE GOAL IN POSITIVE TERMS. Do not use any negative words in your goal statement. For example it is better to say "I enjoy eating healthy, low-calorie, nutritious foods" than "I will not eat sugar, candy, ice cream, and other fattening foods." Remember, always state the goal in positive terms and do not use any negative words in the goal statement.

MAKE YOUR GOAL ATTAINABLE AND REALISTIC. Again, goals can be used to create a success cycle and positive self image. Little things add up to make a major difference in the way you feel about yourself.

BE SPECIFIC. The more clearly your goal is defined, the more likely you are to reach it. For example, if you want to lose weight – What is the weight you desire? What is the body fat percentage or measurements you desire? Clearly define what it is you want to achieve.

STATE THE GOAL IN THE PRESENT TENSE, NOT THE FUTURE TENSE. In order to reach your goal, you have to believe you have already attained it. You must literally program yourself to achieve the goal. See and feel yourself having already achieved the goal and success will be yours. Remember always state your goal in the present tense.

Any voyage begins with one step and is followed by many other steps. Remember to set short-term goals that can be used to help you achieve your long-term goals. Get into the habit of asking yourself the following question each morning and evening: "What must I do today to achieve my long-term goal?"

STEP 6 – PRACTICE POSITIVE VISUALIZATIONS

Positive visualization or imagery is another powerful tool in creating health, happiness, or success. Many believe that we have to be able to see our lives the way we want them to be before it happens. In terms of ideal health, you absolutely must picture yourself in ideal health if you truly want to experience this state. You can use visualization in all areas of your life, but especially for your health. In fact, some of the most promising research on the power of visualization involves enhancing the immune system in the treatment of cancer. Be creative and have fun with positive visualizations and you will soon find yourself living your dreams. It is our dreams that propel us as we roll through this life. They are powerful and inspirational. In fact, the famous author Anatole France said something about dreams and life that really hits home – "existence would be intolerable if we were never to dream."

STEP 7 – LAUGH LONG AND OFTEN

Humor may be the most powerful stress-buster around. By laughing frequently and taking a lighter view of life, you will also find that life is much more enjoyable and fun. Researchers are discovering that laughter enhances the immune system and promotes improved physiology. Recent medical research has also confirmed that laughter:

- Enhances blood flow to the body's extremities and improves cardiovascular function.

- Plays an active part in the body's release of endorphins and other natural mood-elevating and pain-killing chemicals.

- Improves the transfer of oxygen and nutrients to internal organs.

HERE ARE SEVEN TIPS TO HELP YOU GET MORE LAUGHTER IN YOUR LIFE.

TIP 1 **LEARN TO LAUGH AT YOURSELF.** Recognize how funny some of your behavior really is – especially your shortcomings or mistakes. We all have little idiosyncrasies or behaviors that are unique to us that we can recognize and enjoy. Don't take yourself too seriously.

TIP 2 **INJECT HUMOR ANYTIME IT IS APPROPRIATE.** People love to laugh. Get a joke book and learn how to tell a good joke. Humor and laughter really make life enjoyable.

TIP 3 **READ THE COMICS TO FIND ONE THAT YOU FIND FUNNY, AND FOLLOW IT.** Humor is very individual. What I may find funny, you may not, but the comics or "funny papers" have something for everybody. Read them thoroughly to find a comic strip that you find particularly funny and look for it every day or week.

TIP 4 **WATCH COMEDIES ON TELEVISION.** With modern technology, it is amazingly easy to find something funny on television or the internet. When you are in need of a good laugh, try to find something that you can laugh at on TV or YouTube. Some of my favorites are the old-time classics like Andy Griffith, Gilligan's Island, Mary Tyler Moore, etc.

TIP 5 **GO TO COMEDIES AT THE MOVIE THEATER.** Most people love to go to the movies and especially enjoy a good comedy. When people see a funny movie together, they find themselves laughing harder and longer than if they had seen the same scene by themselves. We all feed off each other's laughter during and after the movie. Also, laughing together helps build good relationships.

TIP 6   **PLAY WITH KIDS**. Kids really know how to laugh and play. If you do not have kids of your own, spend time with your nieces, nephews, or neighborhood children with whose families you are friendly. Become a Big Brother or Big Sister. Investigate local Little Leagues. Help out at your church's Sunday School and at children's events.

TIP 7   **ASK YOURSELF THE QUESTION – "WHAT IS FUNNY ABOUT THIS SITUATION?"** Many times we will find ourselves in seemingly impossible situations, but, if we can laugh about it, somehow they become enjoyable or at least tolerable experiences. So many times, we hear people say, "This is something that you will look back on and laugh about." Well, why wait – find the humor in the situation and enjoy a good laugh immediately.

CALMING THE MIND AND BODY

Another important step in fighting stress is learning to calm the mind and body. Among the easiest methods to learn are relaxation exercises. The goal of relaxation techniques is to produce a physiological response known as a *relaxation response* – a response that is exactly opposite to the stress response, and which activates the parasympathetic nervous system. Although an individual may relax simply by sleeping, watching television, or reading a book, relaxation techniques are designed specifically to produce the relaxation response.

Relaxation response is a term coined in the early 1970s by Harvard professor and cardiologist, Herbert Benson, to describe a physiological response that he found in people who meditate that is just the opposite of the stress response.[6] With the stress response (Table 2.1), the sympathetic nervous system dominates. It is designed to protect us against immediate danger. As mentioned above, the relaxation response (Table 2.2) activates the parasympathetic nervous system. The parasympathetic nervous system controls bodily functions such as digestion, breathing, and heart rate during periods of rest, relaxation, visualization, meditation, and sleep. Although the sympathetic nervous system is designed to protect against immediate danger, the parasympathetic system is designed for repair, maintenance, and restoration of the body.

The relaxation response can be achieved through a variety of techniques. It doesn't matter which technique you choose, because all techniques have the same physiological effect – a state of deep relaxation. The most popular techniques are meditation, prayer, progressive relaxation, self-hypnosis, and biofeedback. To produce the desired long-term health benefits, the patient should use the relaxation technique for at least 5–10 minutes each day.

Table 2.1 – The Stress Response

- The heart rate and force of contraction of the heart increase to provide blood to areas necessary to respond to the stressful situation.

- Blood is shunted away from the skin and internal organs, except the heart and lungs, while the amount of blood supplying required oxygen and glucose to the muscles and brain is increased.

- The rate of breathing increases to supply necessary oxygen to the heart, brain, and exercising muscle.

- Sweat production increases to eliminate toxic compounds produced by the body, and to lower body temperature.

- Production of digestive secretions is severely reduced because digestive activity is not critical to counteracting stress.

- Blood sugar levels are raised dramatically as the liver dumps stored glucose into the blood stream.

Table 2.2 – The Relaxation Response

- The heart rate is reduced and the heart beats more efficiently. Blood pressure is reduced.

- Blood is shunted towards internal organs, especially those organs involved in digestion.

- The rate of breathing decreases as oxygen demand is reduced during periods of rest.

- Sweat production diminishes, because a person who is calm and relaxed does not experience nervous perspiration.

- Production of digestive secretions is increased, greatly improving digestion.

- Blood sugar levels are maintained in the normal range.

LEARNING HOW TO BREATHE

Producing deep relaxation with any relaxation technique requires learning how to breathe. Have you ever noticed how a baby breathes? With each breath the baby's abdomen rises and falls because the baby is breathing with its diaphragm, a dome-shaped muscle that separates the chest cavity from the abdominal cavity. If you are like most adults, you tend to fill only your upper chest because you do not utilize the diaphragm. Shallow breathing tends to produce tension and fatigue.

One of the most powerful methods of producing less stress and more energy is by breathing with the diaphragm. By using the diaphragm to breathe, a person dramatically changes their physiology. It literally activates the relaxation centers in the brain. Here is a 10-step technique for learning diaphragmatic breathing.

1. Find a comfortable and quiet place to lie down or sit.

2. Place your feet slightly apart. Place one hand on your abdomen near your navel. Place the other hand on your chest.

3. You will be inhaling through your nose and exhaling through your mouth.

4. Concentrate on your breathing. Note which hand is rising and falling with each breath.

5. Gently exhale most of the air in your lungs.

6. Inhale while slowly counting to 4. As you inhale, slightly extend your abdomen, causing it to rise about 1 inch. Make sure that you are not moving your chest or shoulders.

7. As you breathe in, imagine the warmed air flowing in. Imagine this warmth flowing to all parts of your body.

8. Pause for 1 second, then slowly exhale to a count of 4. As you exhale, your abdomen should move inward.

9. As the air flows out, imagine all your tension and stress leaving your body.

10. Repeat the process until a sense of deep relaxation is achieved.

PROGRESSIVE RELAXATION

One of the most popular techniques for producing the relaxation response is progressive relaxation. The technique is based on a very simple procedure of comparing tension with relaxation. Many people are not aware of the sensation of relaxation. In progressive relaxation, an individual is taught what it feels like to relax by comparing relaxation with muscle tension.

The basic technique is to contract a muscle forcefully for a period of 1–2 seconds and then give way to a feeling of relaxation in that muscle. The procedure systematically goes through all the muscles of the body, progressively producing a deep state of relaxation. The procedure begins with contracting the muscles of the face and neck, then the upper arms and chest, followed by the lower arms and hands. The process is repeated progressively down the body, from the abdomen through the buttocks, thighs, and calves, to the feet. This whole process is repeated two or three times. This technique is often used in the treatment of anxiety and insomnia.

FINAL COMMENTS

These stress-reducing techniques may seem fairly simplistic, but considerable medical research has demonstrated that significant results are possible when applying them in the treatment of many stress-related illnesses. Do not underestimate the innate healing power of the human body and mind. Employing these exercises to condition your attitude and promote the relaxation response is extremely powerful medicine – with no side effects!

CHAPTER 3

GET A GOOD NIGHT'S SLEEP

In helping my patients deal with stress, anxiety, depression, or low energy levels my first goal was always to try to improve their sleep quality. It's a great quick fix to feeling better. Think of a time in your life where you did not sleep well for a few days. Were you more easily stressed? Maybe you were irritable or easily angered. For sure your energy levels were down and likely your mood was as well. Now, think of a time in your life where you slept fantastic and woke up with an abundance of energy. Undoubtedly the world looked brighter and you dealt with people in a friendlier manner, and probably felt stress free. I realize that if you are reading this book it has probably been a while since you regularly felt this way, but I hope you get my point. Everything is better after a good night's sleep.

Human sleep is perhaps one of the least understood body process, but its value to human health and proper functioning is without question. Sleep is absolutely essential to both the body and mind. Impaired sleep, altered sleep patterns, and sleep deprivation impair mental and physical function. Many health conditions, particularly depression, chronic fatigue syndrome, and fibromyalgia, are either entirely or partially related to sleep deprivation or disturbed sleep.

SLEEP DEPRIVATION IN THE UNITED STATES

Over the course of a year, over one-half of the U.S. population will have difficulty falling asleep. About 33% of the population experiences insomnia on a regular basis with 17% of the population claiming that insomnia is a major problem in their lives. Many use over-the-counter sedative medications to combat insomnia, while others seek stronger prescription medications from their physicians. Each year up to 12.5% of adults in the U.S. receive prescriptions for drugs to help them sleep.

THE PROBLEM WITH SLEEPING PILLS

Most sleeping pills are technically "sedative hypnotics." This specific class of drugs is also widely used to treat anxiety and stress. Examples include:

- Alprazolam (Alprazolam, Xanax)
- Chlordiazepoxide (Librium)
- Diazepam (Valium)
- Eszopiclone (Lunesta)
- Flurazepam (Dalmane)
- Quazepam (Doral)
- Ramelteon (Rozerem)
- Temazepam (Restoril)
- Triazolam (Halcion)
- Zaleplon (Sonata)
- Zolpidem tartrate (Ambien)

All of these drugs are associated with significant risks. Problems with these drugs include the fact that most are highly addictive and very poor candidates for long-term use. Common side effects include dizziness, drowsiness, and impaired coordination. It is important not to drive or engage in any potentially dangerous activities while on these drugs. Alcohol should never be consumed with these drugs and could be fatal.

The most serious side effects of the conventional anti-anxiety drugs relate to their effects on memory and behavior. Because these drugs act in a powerful manner on brain chemistry, significant changes in brain function and behavior can occur. Severe memory impairment and amnesia of events can also occur, as well as nervousness, confusion, hallucinations, bizarre behavior, and extreme irritability and aggressiveness may result. They have also been shown to increase feelings of depression, including suicidal thinking.

THE DARK SIDE OF SLEEPING PILLS

Daniel F. Kripke, M.D., Professor of Psychiatry Emeritus at the University of California of San Diego worked for over 30 years assessing the risk of sleeping pills. His findings are stunning. The most shocking of his findings was that people who take sleeping pills die sooner than people who do not use sleeping pills. Dr. Kripke examined data from a very large study known as the Cancer Prevention Study I (CPSI). In this study, American Cancer Society volunteers gave questionnaires to over 1 million Americans and then determining six years later whether the participants had survived. Dr. Kripke and his colleagues found that 50% more of those who said that they "often" took sleeping pills had died, compared to participants of the same age, sex, and reported health status who "never" took sleeping pills.[7]

To re-examine these risks, the American Cancer Society agreed to ask participants new questions about sleeping pills in a new study, called The Cancer Prevention Study II (CPSII). In 1982, American Cancer Society volunteers gave health questionnaires to 1.1 million new participants. The survival of these people was ascertained in 1988.

In the CPSII, it was again found that people who said that they used sleeping pills had significantly higher mortality. Those who reported taking sleeping pills 30 or more times per month had 25% greater mortality than those who said that they took no sleeping pills. Those that took sleeping pills just a few times per month showed a 10–15% increase in mortality, compared to those who took no sleeping pills. Sleeping pills appeared unsafe in any amount.[7]

Deaths from common causes such as heart disease, cancer, and stroke were all increased among sleeping pill users. In addition, though the risk was small, daily use of sleeping pills increased the suicide risk by seven times in men and two times in women.

As of 2008, 15 population studies from Scandinavia to Japan have found that the use of sleeping pills showed increased mortality risk.[8] Three of these studies specifically found that the use of sleeping pills predicted increased risk of death from cancer.[9] There is preliminary data that sleeping pills can increase the risk of certain cancers.[10] But, the strongest explanation for the increased risk of mortality with sleeping pill use is that it is associated with an increased frequency of depression. Considerable evidence shows that depression is also associated with an increased risk for an early death.

So what does all this data really mean? First, it may mean that the use of sleeping pills is just an indicator of stress, anxiety, insomnia, and depression. In other words, maybe these people were taking sleeping pills because they were really stressed out and/or depressed, and it was actually the stress or depression that did them in. Or, it could be that the drugs produce complications. For example, it is possible that these drugs interfere with normal sleep repair mechanisms as well as promote depression.

Although all of the benefits of sleep are still a mystery, one of the ways in which sleep recharges the energy within our cells is by removing harmful chemicals from the body (particularly the brain). Sleep functions to enhance antioxidant mechanisms in order to reduce the damage from highly reactive compounds known as free radicals that can damage our cellular components, including our DNA.

DO SLEEPING PILLS IMPAIR SLEEP QUALITY?

Another explanation for the potential negative effects of sleeping pills on longevity is that they actually interfere with normal sleep patterns. From observation of eye movement and brain wave tracings (electroencephalo-graphic [EEG] recordings), sleep is divided into two distinct types: REM (rapid eye movement) sleep and non-REM sleep. During REM sleep the eyes move rapidly and dreaming takes place. When people are awakened during non-REM sleep, they report that they were thinking about everyday matters, but rarely report dreams.

Non-REM sleep is divided into stages 1 through 4 according to the level of brain wave activity and ease of arousal. As sleep progresses there is a deepening of sleep and slower brain wave activity until REM sleep occurs, when suddenly the brain becomes much more active. In adults, the first REM sleep cycle is usually triggered 90 minutes after going to sleep and lasts about 5–10 minutes. After this flurry of activity, brain wave patterns return to those of non-REM sleep for another 90-minute sleep cycle.

Each night most adults experience five or more sleep cycles. REM sleep periods grow progressively longer as sleep continues; the last sleep cycle may produce a REM sleep period that can last about an hour. Non-REM sleep accounts for approximately 50% of this 90-minute sleep cycle in infants and about 80% in adults. As people age, in addition to having less REM sleep, they tend to awaken when they transition from non-REM to REM sleep.

Disturbance of the normal rhythm of sleep as well as an impaired ability to reach the deeper stages (3 and 4) of non-REM sleep have long been known to be a problem with many sedative hypnotic drugs. It's the main reason why these drugs will often produce a morning "hangover" feeling. In contrast, natural sleep enhancers (e.g., melatonin, 5-HTP, L-theanine, etc.) appear to actually increase the time spent in the deeper levels of non-REM sleep allowing for the brain and body to get fully recharged. When I talk about sleep quality, what I am really referring to is spending sufficient time in those deeper levels of sleep. While sleeping pills increase sleeping time, they do not improve sleep quality. And, based upon the population-based studies, they do not appear to improve our health, but actually rob us of it.

Given the problems with these drugs, every effort should be made to avoid their use. Certainly they are not suitable for long-term use for insomnia.

IMPROVING SLEEP QUALITY NATURALLY

Like other health conditions, the most effective ways to improve sleep quality are based upon identifying and addressing factors that impair sleep. For example, let's take a look at the most common form of insomnia – sleep maintenance insomnia. In this form, people are able to get to sleep, but awaken 3, 4 or 5 hours later and have a really tough time getting back to sleep. What I have found is that most people with sleep maintenance insomnia suffer from faulty blood sugar control. Basically, these people are on what I refer to as the "blood sugar roller coaster." New techniques in blood sugar monitoring have shown quite clearly that nighttime fluctuations in blood sugar levels are the major cause of sleep maintenance insomnia. The recommendations given in the next chapter are critical in helping many people with sleep maintenance insomnia get the good night's sleep they need and desire.

Other common causes of insomnia are stress, depression, anxiety, sensitivity to caffeine, and certain medications – there are well over 300 drugs that can interfere with normal sleep. Elimination of the cause is by far the best treatment.

One of the first steps to improving sleep quality in many people is eliminating caffeine. The average American consumes 150–225 mg of caffeine daily, or roughly the amount of caffeine in 1–2 cups of coffee. Although most people can handle this amount, there is a huge – 15-fold – variation in the rate at which people detoxify stimulants such as caffeine. Genetic variation in the liver enzyme that breaks down caffeine means that some people can eliminate caffeine while others have a form that works so slowly

SEVEN ADDITIONAL TIPS FOR A GOOD NIGHT'S SLEEP

Make your bedroom primarily a place for sleeping. It is not a good idea to use your bed for paying bills, doing work, watching TV, etc. Help your body recognize that this is a place for rest or intimacy. Make sure your room is well ventilated and the temperature consistent. And try to keep it quiet. You could use a fan or a "white noise" machine to help block outside noises.

Incorporate bedtime rituals. Listening to soft music or sipping a cup of herbal tea cues your body that it's time to slow down and begin to prepare for sleep. Try to go to bed and wake up at the same time everyday, even on the weekends. Keeping a regular schedule will help your body expect sleep at the same time each day. Don't oversleep to make up for a poor night's sleep – doing that for even a couple of days can reset your body clock and make it hard for you to get to sleep at night.

Relax for a while before going to bed. Spending quiet time can make falling asleep easier. This may include meditation, relaxation and/or breathing exercises, or taking a warm bath. Try listening to recorded relaxation or guided imagery programs.

Get out of bed if unable to sleep. Don't lie in bed awake. Go into another room and do something relaxing until you feel sleepy. Worrying about falling asleep actually keeps many people awake.

Don't do anything stimulating. Don't read anything job related or watch a stimulating TV program (commercials and news shows tend to increase alertness). Don't expose yourself to bright light. The light gives cues to your brain that it is time to wake up.

Perform progressive relaxation. This technique is based on a very simple procedure of comparing tension to relaxation (see page 21 for how to do it).

Consider changing your bedtime. If you are experiencing sleeplessness or insomnia consistently, think about going to bed later so that the time you spend in bed is spent sleeping. If you are only getting five hours of sleep at night, figure out what time you need to get up and subtract five hours (for example, if you want to get up at 6:00 am, go to bed at 1:00 am). This may seem counterproductive and, at first, you may be depriving yourself of some sleep, but it can help train your body to sleep consistently while in bed and hopefully you will be able to gradually start going to bed earlier and still be able to sleep through the night.

it may take them as much as 12–24 hours to fully eliminate the caffeine from a single cup of coffee. Anyone who has trouble sleeping should simply try caffeine avoidance for 7–10 days. This avoidance has to be strict, so all sources, not just coffee, but tea, chocolate, drugs with caffeine, energy drinks, etc. must be avoided.

Alcohol must also be eliminated in people with regular insomnia. Alcohol causes the release of adrenaline and disrupts the production of serotonin (an important brain chemical that initiates sleep). Although not considered a stimulant, sugar and refined carbohydrates can interfere with sleep. Eating a diet high in sugar and refined carbohydrates, and eating irregularly, can cause a reaction in the body that triggers the fight or flight response, causing wakefulness.

NATURAL SLEEP AIDS

There are a number of natural products that can help improve sleep quality. The specific product that I recommend provides a combination of melatonin (3 mg), 5-HTP (30 mg), and L-theanine (200 mg) in a great-tasting chewable tablet or softgel capsule. These three ingredients work together to decrease the time required to get to sleep and to decrease the number of nighttime awakenings. It works extremely well in most people. Here is a brief description of each ingredient as it relates to improving sleep quality. In addition, there will be a brief discussion on the herb valerian.

MELATONIN

The most popular natural aid for sleep is melatonin. Supplementation with melatonin has been shown in several studies to be very effective in helping induce and maintain sleep in both children and adults, and in both people with normal sleep patterns and those with insomnia. However, the sleep-promoting effects of melatonin are most apparent if melatonin levels in the body are low. In other words, using melatonin is not like taking a sleeping pill. It has a sedative effect only when melatonin levels are low. When melatonin is taken just before going to bed in normal subjects or in patients with insomnia who have normal melatonin levels, it produces no sedative effect. This is because there is normally a rise in melatonin secretion just before going to bed. Melatonin supplementation appears to be most effective in treating insomnia in the elderly, in whom low melatonin levels are quite common.[11, 12]

A dose of 3 mg at bedtime is usually enough, because doses as low as 0.1–0.3 mg have been shown to produce a sedative effect when melatonin levels are low.[13] Although melatonin appears to have no serious side effects at recommended doses, melatonin supplementation could conceivably disrupt the normal daily hormonal rhythm (the circadian rhythm). In one study, a dosage of 8 mg/day for only four days resulted in significant alterations in hormone secretions.[14]

5-HTP (5-HYDROXYTRYPTOPHAN)

5-HTP is converted in the brain to serotonin – an important initiator of sleep. It is one step closer to serotonin than L-tryptophan and has shown more consistent results in promoting and maintaining sleep, even though used at lower dosages.[15-18] One of the key benefits of 5-HTP is its ability to increase REM sleep (typically by about 25%), while increasing deep sleep stages 3 and 4 without lengthening total sleep time.[19, 20] The sleep stages that are reduced to compensate for the increases are non-REM stages 1 and 2 – the least important stages. To take advantage of the sleep-promoting effects of 5-HTP, the recommended dosage is 50–150 mg, 30–45 minutes before retiring. Start with the lower dose for at least three days before increasing it if necessary.

L-THEANINE

L-theanine is a unique amino acid found almost exclusively in tea plants (*Camellia sinensis*). Clinical studies have demonstrated that L-theanine reduces stress, improves the quality of sleep, diminishes the symptoms of PMS (premenstrual syndrome), heightens mental acuity and reduces the negative side effects of caffeine.

At typical dosages, e.g., 100–200 mg, L-theanine does not act as a sedative, but it does significantly improve sleep quality.[21] It is an excellent support agent to melatonin and 5-HTP. As described above, these ingredients exert synergistic effects to promote restful sleep. **NOTE:** At higher single dosages, e.g., 600 mg, L-theanine does exert a sedative effect.

VALERIAN

In terms of herbal medicine, there is no question that valerian *(Valeriana officinalis)* is the most popular remedy for insomnia. Recent scientific studies have substantiated valerian's ability to improve sleep quality and relieve insomnia. In a large double-blind study involving 128 subjects, it was shown that an aqueous extract of valerian root improved the subjective ratings for sleep quality and sleep latency (the time required to get to sleep), but left no "hangover" the next morning.[22]

In a follow-up study, valerian extract was shown to significantly reduce sleep latency and improve sleep quality in sufferers of insomnia and was suggested to be as effective in reducing sleep latency as small doses of benzodiazepines (Valium).[22] The difference, however, arises from the fact that these drugs also result in increased morning sleepiness. Valerian, on the other hand, actually reduces morning sleepiness.

As a mild sedative, valerian may be taken at the following dose 30–45 minutes before retiring:

Dried root (or as tea) – 1–2 g
Tincture (1:5) – 4–6 ml (1–1.5 tsp)
Fluid extract (1:1) – 1–2 ml (0.5–1 tsp)
Valerian extract (0.8% valeric acid) – 150–300 mg

If morning sleepiness does occur, reduce the dosage. If the dosage was not effective be sure to eliminate those factors that disrupt sleep, such as caffeine and alcohol, before increasing the dosage.

FINAL COMMENTS

I want to reiterate the importance of identifying and addressing factors that impair sleep, such as caffeine, alcohol, and even sleeping pills. In the next chapter, you will learn more fully how faulty blood sugar control contributes to the stress response and insomnia. Stabilizing blood sugar levels is a key step to improving the health of most people in North America.

If you are taking any prescription sleeping pill and wish to discontinue, you need to work with your physician. In general, discontinuing any drug has to be done gradually – especially with benzodiazepines. Employ all of the general measures given above and use the combination of 5-HTP, melatonin, and L-theanine. After one week reduce the dosage of the sleeping pill by half. Continue at this dosage for two weeks before reducing by half again. Stay on this dosage for a month before finally discontinuing.

CHAPTER 4

STABILIZE BLOOD SUGAR LEVELS

Breakthrough developments in blood sugar monitoring have led to greater understanding of how fluctuations in blood sugar levels lead to feelings of stress, depression, and insomnia. Fortunately, there are now effective natural approaches that produce revolutionary effects in stabilizing blood sugar levels within a narrow range. The results are absolutely phenomenal, not only helping people feel better, but also allowing them safe and effective appetite control. This chapter will be a little more technical than the others, but it will be worth the reading because the payoff is so huge.

UNDERSTANDING BLOOD SUGAR CONTROL

A lack as well as an excess of blood sugar (glucose) in the body can be devastating to body processes. For this reason, the body strives to maintain blood sugar levels within a narrow range through the coordinated efforts of several glands and their hormones.

The body responds to the rise in blood glucose levels after meals by secreting insulin – a hormone produced by the pancreas. Insulin lowers blood glucose by increasing the rate at which glucose is taken up by cells throughout the body. Declines in blood glucose can cause the release of adrenalin and cortisol by the adrenal glands.

INSULIN RESISTANCE AND GLYCEMIC VOLATILITY

Insulin resistance is the greatest threat to the health of most Americans. This statement may sound dramatic, but it is 100% accurate. Insulin resistance is the key underlying factor that leads to weight gain, the inability to lose weight, increased risk for heart disease, and the development of type 2 diabetes.

Insulin resistance is tied to abdominal obesity. If your waist circumference is larger than your hips, there is an extremely strong likelihood that you suffer from insulin resistance. You are not alone: current estimates are that eight out of ten adults in the United States are overweight. In addition to 20 million Americans meeting the criteria for type 2 diabetes, another 60 million suffer from prediabetes – a condition characterized by insulin resistance. In both prediabetes and type 2 diabetes there is plenty of insulin being secreted, it's just not able to do its job.

As fat cells in the abdomen grow in size or number, they secrete a number of biologic products (e.g., resistin) that dampen the effect of insulin, impair glucose utilization in skeletal muscle, and promote glucose (blood sugar) production by the liver. Also important is that as the number and size of fat cells increase, they lead to a reduction in the secretion of compounds that promote insulin action, including a novel protein produced by fat cells known as adiponectin. Adiponectin is not only associated with improved insulin sensitivity, it also has anti-inflammatory activity, lowers triglycerides, and blocks the development of atherosclerosis. The net effect of all of these actions by fat cells in the overweight individual is that they severely stress blood sugar control mechanisms, as well as lead to the development of the major complication of diabetes – atherosclerosis. Because of all of these newly discovered hormones secreted by fat cells, the collective fatty tissue in the body is now considered a member of the hormonal (endocrine) system.

WHAT DOES ALL THIS BIOCHEMISTRY HAVE TO DO WITH STRESS?

With insulin resistance comes blood sugar volatility and that leads to repeated stimulation of the adrenal glands to secrete adrenalin and cortisol – mirroring the effects of the fight or flight response. Elevated cortisol levels are not only associated with increased feelings of stress, but also with loss of appetite control, cravings for sugar, and weight gain. Using new technology that allows for continuous monitoring of blood sugar levels, Michael R. Lyon, M.D., has discovered that most people with weight problems and insulin resistance go through their days with remarkably fluctuating blood sugar levels. Dr. Lyon is the Medical and Research Director at the Canadian Centre for Functional Medicine as well as an Adjunct Professor at the University of British Columbia's Food, Nutrition and Health Program.

Dr. Lyon and I have defined these fluctuating blood sugar levels as "increased glycemic volatility," but most often we refer to it as being on the blood sugar roller coaster. Increased glycemic volatility is not only at the heart of most weight problems, it can also be a major factor in reducing our ability to cope with stress. Rapidly fluctuating blood sugar levels are generally a result of more-than-moderate consumption of foods with a high content of refined or simple sugars.

ARE YOU RIDING THE BLOOD SUGAR ROLLER COASTER?

DO ANY OF THE FOLLOWING APPLY TO YOU?

- My waist circumference is larger than my hips.
- It is difficult for me to lose weight.
- I crave sweets.
- I feel much better after I eat.
- I am very irritable if I miss a meal.
- I often cry for no reason.
- Sometimes I feel a bit spacey and disconnected.
- I have elevated blood sugar or triglyceride levels.
- I get anxious for no apparent reason.
- I wake up often during the night.
- I feel hungry all of the time.
- I often get very sleepy in the afternoon.

THE NEGATIVE EFFECTS OF EXCESS CORTISOL

To fully appreciate the effect of excessive cortisol secretion on our physiology, let's take a look at the well-known side effects of a drug form of cortisol, called prednisone. Used primarily in allergic and inflammatory conditions like asthma and rheumatoid arthritis, prednisone is by far the most prescribed oral corticosteroid. It blocks many key steps in the allergic and inflammatory response, including the production and secretion by the white blood cells of compounds that promote inflammation. This disruption of the normal defense functions of the white blood cells is great at stopping the inflammatory response, but it essentially cripples the immune system. Long-term use of prednisone also causes abdominal obesity, puffiness of the face ("moon face"), and accumulation of fat in the upper back ("buffalo hump").

Common side effects of long-term prednisone use at higher dosage levels include: depression; insomnia; mood swings; personality changes and even psychotic behavior; high blood pressure; diabetes; peptic ulcers; acne; excessive facial hair in women; muscle cramps and weakness; thinning and weakening of the skin; osteoporosis; and susceptibility to the formation of blood clots. Unfortunately, every single one of prednisone's side effects, both short and long term, can also occur in our bodies as a result of excessive cortisol secretion.

Cortisol excess is almost always associated with weight gain. Not only does cortisol signal the brain to eat more, it increases the amount of visceral (abdominal) fat.

CORTISOL, MOOD, AND SLEEP

Many of the detrimental effects of cortisol on appetite, mood, and sleep are the result of lowering brain serotonin levels. Serotonin is an important brain chemical that promotes a sense of relaxation and positive mood (happiness). When your brain is low in serotonin, carbohydrate cravings result. What the brain is trying to accomplish by signaling a carbohydrate craving is increasing the manufacture of serotonin from the amino acid tryptophan. Tryptophan has a difficult time getting into the brain because it competes with other amino acids for transport across the blood brain barrier. Thanks to insulin, after a high-carbohydrate meal there are fewer amino acid molecules circulating in the bloodstream to compete with tryptophan. While insulin's primary job is to remove sugar from the blood and help it pass into the cells, it also promotes the absorption of certain amino acids into muscle tissue. As a result, there are fewer amino acids competing with tryptophan for transport through the blood-brain barrier. Therefore, as long as a person has either insulin resistance or high cortisol levels it will lead to low brain serotonin levels, which may result in strong carbohydrate cravings, depression, or insomnia.

CONTINUOUS GLUCOSE MONITORING – A CLOSER LOOK

The Continuous Glucose Monitoring System (CGMS) is an electronic diagnostic system that requires the insertion of a small sensor under the skin of the abdomen. The sensing unit contains a miniaturized electronic device that measures blood sugar and transmits the results every few seconds to a pager-sized computer module worn on the patient's belt for up to one week. The blood sugar measurements can then be downloaded to the doctor's computer.

Using the CGMS, Dr. Lyon was the first to document something that has generally been widely accepted – that most people with weight problems go through their days with tremendous fluctuations in their blood sugar levels. When Dr. Lyon and I started working with people with type 2 diabetes we discovered that stabilizing blood sugar levels was not only the key to improving their diabetes, but also a safe and effective weight loss method. When we began using a newly developed dietary fiber matrix known as PGX® (short for PolyGlycopleX®) our type 2 diabetes patients began telling us that for the first time in their lives they did not feel hungry all the time. As a result, they started consuming fewer calories and weight loss was nearly effortless. Because of our success in helping these patients lose weight, we developed a weight loss strategy – the Hunger Free Forever program – designed to help people successfully lose weight and keep it off. (For more information, go to pgx.com or hungerfreeforever.com).

STABILIZING BLOOD SUGAR LEVELS IS A KEY TO STRESS MANAGEMENT

Dr. Lyon and I found that stabilizing blood sugar levels with the help of PGX® not only assisted people with weight loss, but it had an incredible ability to help people handle stress more effectively. One of the first benefits many people with blood sugar volatility noticed when they started our program was complete relief from insomnia – particularly sleep maintenance insomnia. Remember that a dip in blood glucose levels during the night is an important cause of sleep maintenance insomnia. Improving sleep quality alone may be a key reason why people on the program were better able to deal with stress, but we feel the greatest benefits are probably the result of lowered cortisol levels. We believe that science will eventually confirm that with increased blood sugar volatility comes increased cortisol volatility. By stabilizing blood sugar we are best able to lower cortisol levels by eliminating the major stimulus for cortisol secretion: rapid drops in blood sugar levels.

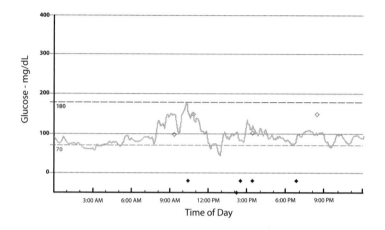

Figure 4.1 – Continuous blood glucose monitoring graph over 24 hours of a typical overweight, nondiabetic patient before starting the Hunger Free Forever program. The patient has elevated glycemic volatility (she is on the blood sugar roller coaster). Monitoring for several days showed that this was her consistent pattern even when she ate healthy food. Frequent food cravings were reported to occur at times that corresponded with when blood sugar rapidly dropped over short periods of time. The black diamonds represent times when the patient feels hungry and then responds by eating. Each time represents an episode of rapidly dropping blood sugar, but only two occasions (while awake) are actual hypoglycemic episodes (below 70 mg/dL). Elevated glycemic volatility with rapid drops in blood sugar explains most "food cravings" or "hunger pangs."

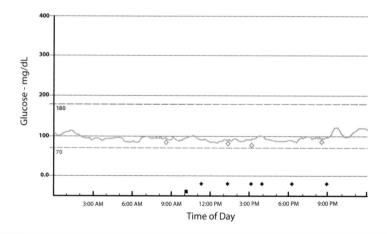

Figure 4.2 – Continuous glucose graph over 24 hours in same patient four weeks into the Hunger Free Forever program. The patient now has nearly normalized glycemic volatility. Appetite and food cravings have dramatically diminished. As well, the patient has more energy and mental clarity. This type of change is very typical with the Hunger Free Forever program and it dramatically illustrates the remarkable changes that can occur.

PGX® IS THE KEY

The ability to stabilize blood sugar levels with the Hunger Free Forever program is the result of using PGX®. This completely new and unique fiber matrix is produced from natural soluble fibers using a patented process that causes these fibers to bind together in a way that makes PGX® the most viscous and soluble fiber ever discovered. And, what that means is that all of the health benefits linked to soluble dietary fibers – including stabilizing blood sugar levels – are significantly magnified with PGX®. Detailed analysis has shown that PGX® produces a higher level of viscosity (gel-forming properties) and expansion with water than the same quantity of any other fiber.[24, 25]

PGX® is able to bind hundreds of times its weight in water, resulting in a volume and viscosity 3–5 times greater than other highly soluble fibers like psyllium or oat beta-glucan (the key fiber in oat bran). To put this in perspective, a small, 5 g serving of PGX® in a meal replacement formula or on its own produces as much volume and viscosity as at least four bowls of oat bran. This means that small quantities of PGX® added to foods or drinks before meals will have an impact on appetite and blood sugar control equivalent to eating enormous and impractical quantities of any other form of fiber.

Detailed clinical studies published in major medical journals and presented at the world's major diabetes conferences have shown PGX® to exert the following benefits:[26-30]

- Balances blood sugar levels in the overweight and obese.

- Reduces appetite and promotes effective weight loss, even in the morbidly obese.

- Increases the level of compounds that block appetite and promote satiety.

- Decreases the level of compounds that stimulate overeating.

- Reduces postprandial (after-meal) blood sugar levels when added to or taken with foods.

- Reduces the glycemic index of any food or beverage.

- Increases insulin sensitivity and decreases blood insulin.

- Improves diabetes control and dramatically reduces the need for insulin or other diabetes medications.

- Lowers total and LDL blood cholesterol and triglycerides.

- In addition, as I mentioned above, we feel that PGX® is an ideal tool for reducing unwanted spikes in cortisol secretion.

HOW TO USE PGX®

PGX® works best if it is used with a low glycemic diet (discussed below). The dosage of PGX® is based on your needs. If you don't need to lose weight and simply want to take advantage of the ability of PGX® to stabilize blood sugar levels, the dosage is only 750–1,500 mg before meals. However, if you want to lose weight, then the dosage needs to be at least 2.5–5 g before meals (start with a dosage of 750–1,000 mg and work your way up to the full dosage over the course of a couple of weeks).

PGX® is available in a variety of different forms: softgel capsules, a zero-calorie drink mix, granules that can be added to foods and beverages, a meal replacement drink mix containing undenatured whey protein, natural flavors, and sweeteners along with vitamins and minerals (SlimStyles®) and a premeal protein drink mix. It does not matter which form you use, just make sure you get the required amount of PGX® before each meal. And, for weight loss I like to recommend taking another dose of PGX® about an hour after dinner to reduce nighttime eating. Be sure to drink 8 oz (250 ml) of water for each 2.5 g dose. For many people, simply taking PGX® softgels 5–15 minutes before meals with a glass of water is the most convenient way to take PGX®.

Detailed studies in both humans and animals have shown that PGX® is very safe and well-tolerated. There are no specific drug interactions, but it is best to take any medication either an hour before or 2–3 hours after taking PGX®.

For more information on where to buy PGX®, how to use it, or the studies behind it, visit pgx.com. Appendix B also provides answers to some of the common questions about PGX®.

EAT TO SUPPORT BLOOD SUGAR CONTROL

In addition to taking PGX®, it is important to avoid foods that cause a rapid rise in blood sugar levels. One useful tool that tells us what foods to avoid is the glycemic index (GI). It is a numerical scale used to indicate how fast and how high a particular food raises blood sugar levels compared to glucose. Refined sugars, white flour products, and other sources of simple carbohydrates and sugars are quickly absorbed into the bloodstream, causing a rapid rise in blood sugar and severely stressing blood sugar control. So it's important to avoid "junk food" and pay attention to the glycemic index of food that you eat. The table on the next page shows the GI score of some common foods.

Table 4.1 – Classification of Foods by Glycemic Index Scores

FRUITS AND NON-STARCHY VEGETABLES		GRAINS, NUTS, LEGUMES, AND STARCHY VEGETABLES	
Very High	**Medium**	**Very High**	**Medium**
None	Cantaloupe	Refined Sugar	Brown rice
	Grapes	Most cold cereals (e.g., Grape Nuts, Corn Flakes, Raisin Bran, etc.)	Oatmeal
High	Orange		Pasta
Banana	Orange Juice	Rice Cakes	Peas
Raisins	Peach	Granola	Pita Bread
Beets	Pineapple	**High**	Pinto Beans
	Watermelon	Bagel	Rye Bread
Low		Bread (white flour)	Whole grain breads
Apple	Green Beans	Carrots	Yams
Apricot	Green Pepper	Corn	
Asparagus	Lettuce	Granola bar	**Low**
Broccoli	Mushrooms	Kidney Beans	Lentils
Brussels Sprouts	Onions	Muffin (bran)	Nuts
Cauliflower	Plums	Potato	Seeds
Celery	Spinach	Pretzels	
Cherries	Strawberries	White Rice	
Cucumber	Tomato	Tortilla	
Grapefruit	Zucchini		

The GI is quite useful, but since it doesn't tell you how much carbohydrate is in a typical serving of a particular food, another tool is needed. That is where glycemic load (GL) comes in. The glycemic load is a relatively new way to assess the impact of carbohydrate consumption. It takes the glycemic index into account, but gives a more complete picture of the effect that a particular food has on blood sugar levels based on how much carbohydrate you actually eat in a serving. A GL of 20 or more is high, a GL of 11–19 inclusive is medium, and a GL of 10 or less is low. For example, let's take a look at beets, a food with a high GI, but a low GL. Although the carbohydrate in beets has a high GI, there isn't a lot of it, so a typical serving of cooked beets has a glycemic load that is very low, about 5. Thus, as long as you eat a reasonable portion of a low GL food, the impact on blood sugar is acceptable, even if the food has a high GI.

To help you manage your food consumption, I have provided a list of the glycemic index, fiber content, and glycemic load of common foods in Appendix C. In essence, foods that are mostly water (e.g., apple or watermelon), fiber (e.g., beet root or carrot) or air (e.g., popcorn) will not cause a steep rise in your blood sugar even if their GI is high, as long as you exercise moderation in portion sizes. I recommend keeping the glycemic load for any three-hour period below 20.

Table 4.2 – Examples of GI, GL, and Insulin Stress Scores of Selected Foods

Food	GI	GL	Glycemic Impact
Carrots, cooked, ¼ cup	49	1.5	Low
Peach, fresh, 1 large	42	3	Low
Beets, cooked ½ cup	64	3	Low
Watermelon, ½ cup	72	4	Low
Whole wheat bread, 1 slice	69	9.6	Low
Baked potato. medium	93	14	Medium
Brown Rice, cooked, 1 cup	50	16	Medium
Banana, raw, 1 medium	55	17.6	Medium

Spaghetti, white, cooked, 1 cup	41	23	High
White rice, cooked, 1 cup	72	26	High
Grape Nuts®, ½ cup	71	33	Very High
Soft drinks, 375 ml	68	34.7	Very High

FINAL COMMENTS

Obesity has replaced cigarette smoking as the major cause of premature death in America. Each year obesity-related conditions cost over $100 billion in health care expenses and cause an estimated 300,000 premature deaths in the U.S. Obesity is perhaps the most significant threat to the future of the United States, Canada, and other developed nations.

CHAPTER 5

NOURISH YOUR BODY AND BRAIN

Whether stress is harmful or not depends on the strength of our entire biological system. What determines the strength of our body and brain? It can be strongly argued that delivering high quality nutrition to the cells of the body is the critical determining factor.

When the eating habits of Americans as a whole are examined it is little wonder that so many people are suffering from stress, anxiety, and fatigue. Most Americans are not providing the body with the high quality nutrition it deserves. When a machine does not receive the proper fuel or maintenance, how long can it be expected to run in an efficient manner? If your body is not fed the full range of nutrients it needs, how can it be expected to stay in a state of good health?

Instead of eating foods rich in vital nutrients, most Americans focus on refined foods high in calories, sugar, fat, and cholesterol. Instead of eating life-giving foods, Americans are filling up on cheeseburgers, French fries, potato chips, and chocolate chip cookies, and washing them down with artificially colored and flavored fruit drinks or colas. There is no question that one of the easy steps to eating a health-promoting diet is to reduce the intake of potentially harmful substances – foods laden with empty calories, additives, and artificial sweeteners – and replace them with natural foods, preferably organically grown.

KEY DIETARY RECOMMENDATIONS

The most important dietary recommendation for improving stress management – eating to improve blood sugar control – was given in the previous chapter. Here are some additional goals:

- Keep salt intake low, potassium intake high.
- Take a high-potency multiple vitamin and mineral formula.
- Take a pharmaceutical-grade fish oil.

For additional guidance in constructing a health-promoting diet, see the optimal health food pyramid in Appendix E on page 125.

KEEP SALT INTAKE LOW, POTASSIUM INTAKE HIGH

One of the key dietary recommendations to support the adrenal glands is to ensure adequate potassium levels in the body. This can best be done by consuming foods rich in potassium and avoiding foods high in sodium. Most Americans have a dietary potassium-to-sodium (K:Na) ratio of less than 1:2. In contrast, most researchers recommend a dietary K:Na ratio greater than 5:1. However, even this recommendation may not be optimal. A natural diet rich in fruits and vegetables can produce a K:Na ratio greater than 50:1, as most fruits and vegetables have a K:Na ratio of more than 100:1. The average K:Na ratios for several common fresh fruits and vegetables are as follows:

- Carrots: 75:1

- Potatoes: 110:1
- Apples: 90:1
- Bananas: 440:1
- Oranges: 260:1

In the U.S., only 5% of sodium intake comes from the natural ingredients in food. Prepared foods contribute 45% of our sodium intake; 45% is added in cooking; and another 5% is added as condiments. You can reduce your salt intake by following these tips:

1. Take the salt shaker off the table.

2. Omit added salt from recipes and food preparation.

3. To boost your potassium levels use salt substitutes such as NoSalt, Nu-Salt, or Also Salt. These products are made with potassium salts and taste very similar to regular salt (sodium chloride). They can be found in health food stores as well as many mainstream grocery stores.

4. Learn to enjoy the flavors of unsalted foods.

5. Try flavoring foods with herbs, spices, and lemon juice.

6. Read food labels carefully to determine the amounts of sodium. Learn to recognize ingredients that contain sodium. Salt, soy sauce, salt brine, and any ingredient with "sodium" (such as monosodium glutamate) or "baking soda" (sodium bicarbonate) as part of its name contains sodium.

7. In reading labels and menus, look for words that signal high sodium content, such as smoked, barbecued, pickled, broth, soy sauce, teriyaki, Creole sauce, marinated, cocktail sauce, tomato base, Parmesan, and mustard sauce.

8. Do not eat canned vegetables or soups, which are often extremely high in sodium.

9. Choose low-salt (reduced-sodium) products when available.

TAKE A HIGH POTENCY MULTIPLE VITAMIN AND MINERAL FORMULA

Nutritional supplementation – the use of vitamins, minerals, and other food factors to support good health – is an important component of a

EASY TIPS TO INCREASE YOUR INTAKE OF FRUITS AND VEGETABLES

- Buy many kinds of fruits and vegetables when you shop, so you have plenty of choices.

- Stock up on frozen vegetables for easy cooking, so that you always have a vegetable dish with your dinner.

- Use the fruits and vegetables that go bad quickly (peaches, asparagus) first. Save hardier varieties (apples, acorn squash) or frozen goods for later in the week.

- Keep fruits and vegetables where you can see them. The more often you see them, the more likely you are to eat them.

- Keep a bowl of cut-up vegetables on the top shelf of the refrigerator.

- Make up a big tossed salad with several kinds of greens, cherry tomatoes, carrot, red pepper, broccoli, scallions, and sprouts. Refrigerate in a large glass bowl with an air-tight lid, so a delicious mixed salad will be ready to enjoy for several days.

- Keep a fruit bowl on your kitchen counter, table, or desk at work.

- Treat yourself to a fruit sundae. Top a bowl of your favorite cut up fruits with vanilla yogurt, shredded coconut, and a handful of nuts.

- Pack a piece of fruit or some cut-up vegetables in your briefcase or backpack; carry moist towelettes for easy cleanup.

- Add fruits and vegetables to lunch by having them in soup, salad, or cut up raw.

- Use thinly sliced pears or apples in your next omelet.

- At dinner, serve steamed or microwaved vegetables.

- Add fresh greens such as Swiss chard, collards or beet greens to stir fries.

- Choose fresh fruit for dessert. For a special dessert, try a fruit parfait with low-fat yogurt or sherbet topped with lots of berries.

- Add extra varieties of vegetables when you prepare soups, sauces, and casseroles (for example, add grated carrots and zucchinis to spaghetti sauce).

- When dining out, take advantage of salad bars, which offer ready-to-eat raw vegetables and fruits, and prepared salads made with fruits and vegetables.

- Use vegetable-based sauces such as marinara sauce, and drink juices such as low sodium v-8 or tomato juice.

- Freeze lots of blueberries. They make a great summer replacement for ice cream, popsicles, and other sugary treats.

stress management program. The key functions of nutrients like vitamins and minerals in the human body revolve around their role as essential components of enzymes and coenzymes. One of the key concepts in nutritional medicine is to supply the necessary support or nutrients to allow the enzymes of a particular tissue to work at their optimum levels.

In the last few decades more Americans than ever are taking nutritional supplements. Research shows that over half of all Americans take some form of dietary supplement on a regular basis. Why are so many Americans taking supplements? They know they are not getting all that they need from their diets and realize that supplements make them feel healthier. Numerous studies have demonstrated that most Americans consume a diet inadequate in nutritional value. Comprehensive studies sponsored by the U.S. government (e.g., NHANES I, II, III, and 2007–2008; Ten State Nutrition Survey; USDA nationwide food consumption studies, etc.) have revealed that marginal nutrient deficiencies exist in a substantial portion of the U.S. population (approximately 50%) and that in certain age groups more than 80% of the group consumed less than the recommended dietary intake level of certain specified nutrients.

These studies indicate that the chances of consuming a diet supplying the recommended dietary intake (RDI) for all nutrients is extremely unlikely for most Americans. In other words, while it is theoretically possible that a healthy individual can get all the nutrition they need from foods, the fact is that most Americans do not even come close to meeting all their nutritional needs through diet alone. In an effort to increase their intake of essential nutrients, many Americans look to vitamin and mineral supplements.

Multivitamin products – defined as dietary supplements that contain at least three vitamins and may or may not contain minerals – were the most reported supplement in all the NHANES surveys including NHANES 2007–2008. [1]

While most Americans may be deficient in a given vitamin or mineral, the level of deficiency is usually serious enough for obvious nutrient deficiencies to be apparent. A severe deficiency disease like scurvy (severe lack of vitamin C) is extremely rare, but marginal vitamin C deficiency is thought to be relatively common. The term "subclinical deficiency" is often used to describe marginal nutrient deficiencies. A subclinical or marginal deficiency indicates a deficiency of a particular vitamin or mineral that is not severe enough to produce a classic deficiency sign or symptom. In many instances the only clue that there is a subclinical nutrient deficiency may be fatigue, lethargy, difficulty concentrating, a lack of well-being, or some other vague symptom. Worse, however, is that – as we extensively document in this book – chronic, long-term marginal deficiencies are an underlying cause of most of the diseases we suffer from in Western societies. Diagnosis of subclinical deficiencies is an extremely difficult process that involves detailed dietary or laboratory analysis. It's not worth the cost to perform these tests because they are usually far more expensive than taking a year's supply of the vitamin being tested for.

THE RDA IS NOT ENOUGH

Recommended Dietary Allowances (RDAs) for vitamins and minerals have been prepared by the Food and Nutrition Board of the National Research Council since 1941. These guidelines were originally developed to reduce the rates of severe nutritional deficiency diseases such as scurvy (deficiency of vitamin C), pellagra (deficiency of niacin) and beriberi (deficiency of vitamin B_1). In the mid-1990s, these guidelines were replaced by Food and Drug Administration (FDA) nutritional guidelines known as Recommended Daily Intake levels (RDIs). The RDIs show no more promise than the RDAs did in providing the public with useful information on the intake of nutrients for the prevention, mitigation, and treatment of a wide range of conditions and diseases for which diet and specific nutrients may be of benefit.

A tremendous amount of scientific research indicates that the "optimal" level for many nutrients, especially the so-called antioxidant nutrients like vitamins C and E, beta-carotene, and selenium, may be much higher than their current RDI. The RDIs focus only on the prevention of overt nutritional deficiencies in population groups, they do not define "optimal" intake for an individual.

Another factor the RDIs do not adequately take into consideration are environmental and lifestyle factors which can destroy vitamins and bind minerals. For example, even the Food and Nutrition Board acknowledges that smokers require at least twice as much vitamin C as nonsmokers. But what about other nutrients and smoking? And what about the effects of alcohol consumption, food additives, heavy metals (lead, mercury, etc.), carbon monoxide, and other chemicals associated with our modern society that are known to interfere with nutrient function? Dealing with the hazards of modern living may be another reason why many people take supplements.

While the RDIs have done a good job of defining the minimum nutrient levels needed to prevent nutritional deficiencies, there is still much to be learned regarding the optimal nutrient levels.

KEY NUTRIENTS TO PROTECT AGAINST STRESS

Several nutrients are especially important in protecting against the effects of stress – vitamin C, vitamin B_6, zinc, magnesium, and pantothenic acid. All of these nutrients play a critical role in the health of the adrenal gland as well as the manufacture of adrenal hormones. There is evidence that indicates that during times of stress, the levels of these nutrients in the adrenals can plummet.

For example, it is well known that during times of chemical, emotional, psychological, or physiological stress, the body has an increased need for vitamin C. Examples of chemical stressors include cigarette smoke, pollutants, and allergens. Extra vitamin C in the form of supplementation, along with an increased intake of foods rich in vitamin C, is often recommended to keep the immune system working properly during times of stress.

Equally important during high periods of stress or for individuals needing adrenal support is pantothenic acid (a B vitamin). Pantothenic acid deficiency results in adrenal atrophy (wasting away) characterized by fatigue, headache, sleep disturbances, nausea, and abdominal discomfort. Pantothenic acid is found in whole grains, legumes, cauliflower, broccoli, salmon, liver, sweet potatoes, and tomatoes. In addition, it is a good idea to take at least an additional 100 mg of pantothenic acid daily. The other key nutrients – vitamin B_6, zinc, and magnesium – should be taken at the levels recommended below.

A QUICK GUIDE TO MULTIPLE VITAMIN AND MINERAL FORMULAS

The first thing to look for when selecting a multiple vitamin and mineral formula is to make sure that it provides the full range of vitamins and minerals. There are 13 different known vitamins, each with its own special role to play. The vitamins are classified into two groups: fat soluble (vitamins A, D, E, and K) and water soluble (the B vitamins and vitamin C). Vitamins function along with enzymes in chemical reactions necessary for human bodily function, including energy production. Together, vitamins and enzymes work together to act as catalysts in speeding up the making or breaking of chemical bonds that join molecules together.

There are 22 different minerals important in human nutrition. Minerals function, along with vitamins, as components of body enzymes. Minerals are also needed for proper composition of bone and blood, and maintaining normal cell function.

Taking a high-quality multiple vitamin and mineral supplement providing all of the known vitamins and minerals serves as a foundation upon which to build a nutritional supplementation program. Dr. Roger Williams, one of the premier biochemists of our time, states that healthy people should use multiple vitamin and mineral supplements as an "insurance formula" against possible deficiency. This does not mean that a deficiency will occur in the absence of the vitamin and mineral supplement, any more than not having fire insurance means that your house will burn down. But given the enormous potential for individual differences from person to person, and the varied mechanisms of vitamin and mineral actions, supplementation with a multiple formula seems to make sense. The following recommendations provide an optimum intake range to guide you in selecting a high-quality multiple vitamin and mineral supplement.

Vitamins	Daily Dose for Adults and Children 9 or More Years of Age
Vitamin A (retinol) [a]	2,500–5,000 IU
Vitamin A (from beta-carotene)	5,000–25,000 IU
Vitamin B_1 (thiamin)	10–100 mg
Vitamin B_2 (riboflavin)	10–50 mg
Vitamin B_3 (niacin)	10–100 mg
Vitamin B_5 (pantothenic acid)	25–100 mg
Vitamin B_6 (pyridoxine)	25–100 mg
Vitamin B_{12} (methylcobalamin)	400 mcg
Vitamin C (ascorbic acid) [b]	250–1,000 mg
Vitamin D [c]	1,000–2,000 IU
Vitamin E (mixed tocopherols) [d]	100–200 IU
Vitamin K_1 or K_2	60–300 mcg
Niacinamide	10–30 mg
Biotin	100–300 mcg
Folic acid	400 mcg
Choline	10–100 mg
Inositol	10–100 mg

Minerals	Range for Adults and Children 4 or More Years of Age
Boron	1–6 mg
Calcium [e]	600–1,000 mg
Chromium [f]	200–400 mcg
Copper	1–2 mg

Iodine	50–150 mcg
Iron [g]	15–30 mg
Magnesium	250–500 mg
Manganese	3–5 mg
Molybdenum	10–25 mcg
Potassium	not applicable [h]
Selenium	100–200 mcg
Silica	1–25 mg
Vanadium	50–100 mcg
Zinc	15–30 mg

Notes

a   Women of childbearing age who may become pregnant should not take more than 2,500 IU of retinol daily due to the possible risk of birth defects.

b   It may be easier to take vitamin C separately to achieve the recommended level.

c   Elderly people in nursing homes living in northern latitudes should supplement with vitamin D at the high end of the range.

d   It may be more cost-effective to take vitamin E separately rather than as a component of a multiple vitamin formula.

e   Women who have or who are at risk of osteoporosis may need to take a separate calcium supplement to achieve the recommended level of 1,000 mg daily.

f   For diabetes and weight loss, doses of 600 mcg of chromium can be used.

g   Most men, as well as most women who have gone through menopause, rarely need supplemental iron.

h   The FDA restricts the amount of potassium in supplements to no more than 99 mg. Potassium is not an important mineral in a multiple vitamin and mineral formula; potassium needs are best met through diet and the use of potassium salts used as salt substitutes.

Read labels carefully to find multiple vitamin and mineral formulas that contain doses in these ranges. Be aware that you will not find a formula that provides all of these nutrients at these levels in one single pill – it would simply be too big. Usually you'll need to take at least 3–6 tablets per day to meet these levels. While many "one-a-day" supplements provide good levels of vitamins, they tend to be insufficient in the amount of some of the minerals they provide. Your body needs the minerals as much as the vitamins – the two work hand-in-hand.

Multiple vitamin and mineral supplements are best taken with meals. Whether you take them at the beginning or the end of a meal is up to you. If you are taking more than a couple of pills, you may find that taking them at the beginning of a meal is more comfortable. Taking a handful of pills on a full stomach may cause a little stomach upset.

TAKE A PHARMACEUTICAL-GRADE FISH OIL

One of the major advances in nutritional medicine is the ability to produce a fish oil supplement that is a highly concentrated form of long-chain omega-3 fatty acids and also free from lipid peroxides, heavy metals, environmental contaminants, and other harmful compounds. These "pharmaceutical-grade" fish oil concentrates are so superior to earlier fish oil products that they are literally revolutionizing nutritional medicine because of the health benefits they produce.

While most Americans eat way too much of the omega-6 oils found in meats and most vegetable oils, they suffer a relative deficiency of the omega-3 oils – a situation that is associated with an increased risk for heart disease and about 60 other conditions, including cancer, arthritis, stroke, high blood pressure, skin diseases, and diabetes. Particularly important to good health are the longer chain omega-3 fatty acids eicosapentaenoic acid (EPA) and docosahexaenoic acid (DHA) found in fish, especially cold-water fish such as salmon, mackerel, herring, and halibut, as well as in fish oil supplements.

Why are the long-chain omega-3 fatty acids so important? The answer has to do with the function of these fatty substances in cellular membranes and inflammation. A diet that is deficient in omega-3 fatty acids, particularly EPA and DHA, results in altered cell membranes. Without healthy membranes, cells lose their ability to hold water, vital nutrients, and electrolytes. They also lose their ability to communicate with other cells and to be controlled by regulating hormones. They simply do not function properly. Cell membrane dysfunction is a critical factor in the development of virtually every chronic disease, especially cancer, diabetes, arthritis, and heart disease. Not surprisingly, long-chain omega-3 fatty acids have shown tremendous protective effects against all of these diseases.

Because the brain is the richest source of fats in the human body and proper nerve cell function is critically dependent on proper membrane fluidity, alterations in membrane fluidity affect behavior, mood, and mental function. Studies have shown that the physical properties of brain cell membranes, including fluidity, directly influence the action of brain neurotransmitters and can lead to depression, anxiety, and other psychological disturbances.

Table 5.1 – Some conditions that benefit significantly from fish oil supplementation

---

- Allergies

- Alzheimer's disease

- Arthritis

- Asthma

- Attention deficit disorder

- Autoimmune diseases (e.g., rheumatoid arthritis, lupus, MS, etc.)

- Cancer (both for prevention and as an adjunct to primary treatment)

- Depression

- Diabetes

- Eczema

- Elevated triglyceride levels

- Heart disease (prevention and treatment)

- High blood pressure

- Inflammatory conditions (e.g., ulcerative colitis, Crohn's disease)

- Macular degeneration

- Menopause

- Osteoporosis

- Pregnancy

- Psoriasis

OMEGA-3 FATTY ACIDS IN ANXIETY AND DEPRESSION

For the reasons described above, anxiety and depression are strongly linked to lower levels of omega-3 fatty acids.[31] In addition to being influenced by alterations in cell membrane function, both depression and anxiety can enhance the production of pro-inflammatory compounds known as cytokines. A high intake of omega-6 fatty acids found in corn-fed animal products, dairy, and common vegetable oils like corn, soy, safflower, and sunflower, combined with a low intake of omega-3 fatty acids, can amplify the production of these cytokines. Cytokines not only promote inflammation, but they appear to impact the way we feel as well. So increasing the intake of omega-3 fatty acids and lowering the intake of omega-6 fatty acids may help to reduce anxiety and depression. The positive results with fish oil supplements in clinical depression are well documented. In regards to anxiety and fish oils, preliminary studies have yielded impressive results. In one study, fish oil supplementation decreased feelings of anger and anxiety in substance abusers.[32] In a detailed study involving medical students, 2.5 g daily of long-chain omega-3 fatty acids (2,085 mg EPA and 348 mg DHA) from fish oils showed a 14% decrease in cytokine production and a 20% reduction in anxiety symptoms.[33]

Flaxseed oil, a source of the short-chain omega-3 fatty acid alpha-linolenic acid, also has anti-anxiety effects. In one study, three out of four patients with a long history of agoraphobia improved within 2–3 months after taking flaxseed oil at a dosage of 2–6 tbsp daily, in divided doses, depending upon their response.[34] All patients had signs of essential fatty acid deficiency, such as dry skin, dandruff, brittle fingernails that grow slowly, and nerve disorders.

DOSAGE RECOMMENDATIONS

When selecting a fish oil supplement, it is essential to use a brand that you trust. Rigorous quality control is an absolute must to insure the product is free from heavy metals like lead and mercury, pesticides, damaged fats (lipid peroxides), and other contaminants. For general health, the recommended dosage is 1,000 mg of EPA/DHA daily. Read the label carefully to differentiate between the amount of fish oil and the amount of the EPA and DHA, as the recommendation is not 1,000 mg of fish oil, but 1,000 mg of EPA/DHA. For therapeutic purposes, such as reducing inflammation or lowering triglyceride levels, the dosage recommendation is usually 3,000 mg EPA/DHA daily.

In addition to taking a high quality fish oil, it is also a good idea to take a tbsp of flaxseed oil daily. Flaxseed oil is unique because it contains both omega-3 and omega-6 essential fatty acids – alpha-linolenic acid (omega-3) and linoleic acid (omega-6) – in appreciable amounts. The best way to take flaxseed oil is by adding it to food. Flaxseed oil by the tablespoon is not very palatable. Do not cook with flaxseed oil; use olive or canola oil instead. Because flaxseed oil is easily damaged by heat and light, you must add it to foods after they have been cooked. Here are some suggestions: use it as a salad dressing, dip your bread into it, add it to hot or cold cereal, or spray it over your popcorn. Here is a sample salad dressing featuring flaxseed oil:

BASIC FLAXSEED OIL SALAD DRESSING

Place all ingredients into a salad bowl and whisk together until smooth and creamy. This recipe is quick and delicious!

- 4 tbsp organic flaxseed oil
- 1½ tbsp lemon juice
- 1 medium garlic clove, crushed
- Pinch of seasoned salt or salt-free seasoning
- Fresh ground pepper to taste

Jazz up this basic recipe to your own personal taste by using your favorite herbs and spices.

FINAL COMMENTS

Humans plan; animals act on impulse. One of the principal reasons why weight problems have become so prevalent is that our fast-paced way of life leads us to act on our animal instincts when it comes to food. But eating on impulse often leads to poor dietary choices. Even the busiest people can find the time to do a bit of planning and add some structure to their eating habits. It is important to develop a strategy for meal planning. For example, sit down before the week begins and plan out when, what, and where you are going to eat for the week. If you prepare your own meals, a simple menu plan with seven breakfasts, lunches and dinners along with healthy snacks, can be easily accomplished in about 10–15 minutes. From this menu plan, a grocery list can easily be compiled.

CHAPTER 6

MANAGE YOUR LIFE

Develop a stress-free life does not mean retreating to a cave or a deserted island. While many people do find that simplifying their lives significantly reduces stress, the reality for most is that due to a number of factors (e.g., responsibilities, financial commitments, values, interests, etc.) running away from the stress of modern life is just not possible (or appealing). What can help reduce stress in addition to the methods discussed in previous chapters is learning to manage your life. By "managing your life" I mean actually developing a daily plan and long-term strategy to achieve your goals.

Planning out your day is something that you should do every day, either in the evening of the previous day, or first thing in the morning. Doing so can help you keep your life on course. It reduces stress to know what tomorrow is going to be like. Of course an unexpected event can derail even the best laid plan, but in general it is what we do day in and day out that determines the direction and quality of our lives.

THE IMPORTANCE OF TIME MANAGEMENT

One of the biggest stressors for most people is time. They simply do not feel they have enough of it. Here are seven tips on time management that really seem to work. And by the way, time management does not mean squeezing more and more tasks into less and less time. It means learning to plan out your time more effectively, and allowing time for other activities in life that you enjoy.

ORGANIZE YOUR DAY. There are always interruptions and unplanned demands on your time, but create a definite plan for the day and be sure to include all of the important health habits like menu planning, time for exercise and relaxation exercises, and socializing.

SET PRIORITIES. Realize that you can only accomplish so much in a day. Decide what is important, and limit your efforts to those goals.

DELEGATE AUTHORITY. Delegate as much authority and work as you can. You can't do everything yourself. Learn to train and depend on others.

TACKLE THE TOUGH JOB FIRST EACH DAY. Handle the most important tasks first, while your energy levels are high. Leave the busywork or running around for later in the day.

MINIMIZE MEETING TIME. Schedule meetings to bump up against lunch hour or quitting time; that way they can't last forever.

AVOID PUTTING THINGS OFF. Work done under the pressure of an unreasonable deadline often has to be redone. That creates more stress than if it had been done right the first time. Plan ahead.

DON'T BE A PERFECTIONIST. Do your best in a reasonable amount of time, then move on to other important tasks. If you find time, you can always come back later and polish the task some more.

STRESS AND RELATIONSHIPS

Another major cause of stress for many people is their interpersonal relationships at home, with family and friends, and on the job. Humans are social beings. We need to relate to each other to nourish our mind and soul. However, the reality is that relationships as well as lack of relationships can be a significant source of stress.

The quality of any relationship ultimately comes down to the quality of the communication. Learning to communicate effectively goes a very long way in reducing the stress and occasional (or frequent) conflicts of interpersonal relationships. Here are seven tips to effective communication, regardless of the type of interpersonal relationship:

1. **THE FIRST KEY TO SUCCESSFUL COMMUNICATION IS TO LEARN TO BE A GOOD LISTENER.** Allow the person you are communicating with to really share their feelings and thoughts uninterrupted. Empathize with them; put yourself in their shoes. If you first seek to understand, you will find yourself being better understood.

2. **BE AN ACTIVE LISTENER.** This means that you must actually be engaged and interested in what the other person is communicating. Listen to what they are saying instead of thinking about your response. Ask questions to gain more information or clarify what they are telling you. Good questions encourage better communication.

3. **BE A REFLECTIVE LISTENER.** Restate or reflect back to the other person your interpretation of what they are telling you. This simple technique shows the other person that you are both listening and understanding what they are saying. Restating what you think is being said may cause some short-term conflict in some situations, but it is certainly worth the risk.

4. **WAIT TO SPEAK.** Don't interrupt; wait until the person or people you

want to communicate with are done speaking. If they are not ready to listen, no matter how well you communicate, your message will not be heard.

5. **DON'T TRY TO TALK OVER THE OTHER PERSON.** If you find yourself being interrupted, relax; don't try to out-talk the other person. If you are courteous and allow them to speak, eventually (unless they are extremely rude) they will respond likewise. If they don't, point out to them that they are interrupting the communication process by not reciprocating. You can only do this if you have been a good listener. Double standards in relationships seldom work.

6. **HELP THE OTHER PERSON BECOME AN ACTIVE LISTENER.** This can be done by asking them if they understood what you were communicating. Ask them to tell you what they understood you to say. If they don't seem to understand what it is you are saying, keep at it until they do.

7. **DON'T BE AFRAID OF LONG SILENCES.** Human communication involves much more than spoken words. A great deal can be communicated during silences. Unfortunately in many situations silence can make us feel uncomfortable. Relax. Some people need silence to collect their thoughts and feel safe in communicating. The important thing to remember during silences is that you must remain an active listener.

DEVELOP HEALTH HABITS

The importance of attitude, sleep, diet, supplementation, time management, and relationships has hopefully been stressed sufficiently. Woven together, these things construct our lifestyle and daily habits. There is one other very important item that has only been mentioned in passing. Do you know what it is? Of course you do – its physical exercise. Exercise is a vital component of a comprehensive stress management program and overall good health. The immediate effect of exercise is stress on the body, however, with a regular exercise program the body adapts. The body's response to this regular stress is that it becomes stronger, functions more efficiently, and has greater endurance.

The physical benefits from regular exercise are largely the result of improved cardiovascular and respiratory function. Simply stated, exercise enhances the transport of oxygen and nutrients into cells. At the same time, exercise enhances the transport of carbon dioxide and waste products from the tissues of the body to the blood stream and ultimately out of the body.

Regular exercise is particularly important in reducing the risk of heart disease. It does this by lowering cholesterol levels, improving blood and oxygen supply to the heart, increasing the functional capacity of the heart, reducing blood pressure, reducing obesity, and exerting a favorable effect on blood clotting.

Regular exercise increases stamina and energy levels. People who exercise regularly are much less likely to suffer from fatigue and depression.

THE ANTI-STRESS BENEFITS OF REGULAR EXERCISE

Tensions, depression, feelings of inadequacy, and worries diminish greatly with regular exercise. Regular exercise also exerts a powerfully positive effect on mood. Exercise alone has been demonstrated to have a tremendous impact on mood and the ability to handle stressful life situations.

Participation in exercise, sports, and physical activities is strongly associated with decreased symptoms of anxiety (restlessness, tension, etc.), depression (feeling that life is not worthwhile, low spirits, etc.), and malaise (a run-down feeling, insomnia, etc.).[35] Simply stated, people who participate in regular exercise have higher self-esteem and are happier.

Regular exercise has been shown to increase the amount of powerful mood-elevating substances in the brain known as endorphins. These compounds exert similar effects to morphine, although much milder. In fact, their name (endo = endogenous, -rphins = morphines) was given to them because of their morphine-like mood-enhancing effects. There is a clear association between exercise and endorphin elevation, and when endorphins go up, mood follows.

If the benefits of exercise could be put into a pill, you would have the most powerful health-promoting medication available. Take a look at this long list of health benefits produced by regular exercise:

Table 6.1 – Health Benefits of Regular Exercise

MUSCULOSKELETAL SYSTEM	
Increases muscle strength	Produces stronger bones, ligaments, and tendons
Increases flexibility of muscles and range of joint motion	Enhances posture, poise, and physique
Produces stronger bones, ligaments, and tendons	Improves balance
HEART AND BLOOD VESSELS	
Lowers resting heart rate	Improves oxygen delivery throughout the body
Strengthens heart function	Increases blood supply to muscles
Lowers blood pressure	Enlarges the arteries to the heart
BODILY PROCESSES	
Improves the way the body handles dietary fat	Prevents osteoporosis
Reduces heart disease risk	Improves immune function
Helps lower blood cholesterol and triglycerides	Aids digestion and elimination
Raises HDL, the "good" cholesterol	Increases endurance and energy levels
Helps improve calcium deposition in bones	Promotes lean body mass, burns fat
MENTAL PROCESSES	
Provides a natural release for pent-up feelings	Improves the ability to handle stress
Helps reduce tension and anxiety	Stimulates improved mental function
Improves mental outlook and self-esteem	Encourages relaxation, and improves sleep
Helps relieve moderate depression	Increases self-esteem
LONGEVITY	
Increased life expectancy	

CREATING AN EFFECTIVE EXERCISE ROUTINE

Exercise is clearly one of the most powerful medicines available. Unfortunately, there's no pill. But the time you spend exercising is a valuable investment towards good health. To help you develop a successful exercise program, here are seven steps to follow.

STEP 1 – REALIZE THE IMPORTANCE OF PHYSICAL EXERCISE

The first step is realizing just how important it is to get regular exercise. We cannot stress enough just how vital regular exercise is to your health. But, as much as we stress this fact it means absolutely nothing unless it really sinks in and you accept it. You must make regular exercise a top priority in your life.

STEP 2 – CONSULT YOUR PHYSICIAN

If you are not currently on a regular exercise program, get medical clearance if you have health problems or if you are over 40 years of age. The main concern is the functioning of your heart. Exercise can be quite harmful (and even fatal) if your heart is not able to meet the increased demands placed on it.

It is especially important to see a physician if you have any of the following symptoms:

- Heart disease
- Smoking
- High blood pressure
- Extreme breathlessness with physical exertion
- Pain or pressure in the chest, arm, teeth, jaw or neck when you exercise
- Dizziness or fainting
- Abnormal heart action (palpitations or irregular heart beat)

STEP 3 – SELECT AN ACTIVITY YOU CAN ENJOY

If you are fit enough to begin, the next thing to do is to select an activity that you feel you would enjoy. Using the list below, choose from one to five of the activities – or fill in a choice or two of your own – that you think you might enjoy. Make a commitment to do one activity a day for at least 20 minutes, and preferably an hour. Make your goal the enjoyment of the activity. The important thing is to move your body enough to raise your pulse a bit above its resting rate.

The best exercises for your heart are the kind that elevate your heart rate the most. Aerobic activities such as walking briskly, jogging, bicycling, cross-country skiing, swimming, aerobic dance, and racquet sports are good examples. Brisk walking (five miles an hour) for approximately 30 minutes may be the very best form of exercise for weight loss. Walking can be done anywhere. It doesn't require any expensive equipment, just comfortable clothing and well-fitting shoes, and the risk of injury is extremely low. If you decide to walk on a regular basis, I strongly urge you to purchase a pair of high-quality walking or jogging shoes.

STEP 4 – MONITOR EXERCISE INTENSITY

Exercise intensity is determined by measuring your heart rate (the number of times your heart beats per minute). This determination can be quickly done by placing the index and middle finger of one hand on the side of the neck just below the angle of the jaw or on the opposite wrist. Beginning with zero, count the number of heartbeats for six seconds. Simply add a zero to this number and that is your pulse. For example, if you counted 14 beats, your heart rate would be 140. Would this be a good number? It depends upon your "training zone."

A quick and easy way to determine your maximum training heart rate is simply to subtract your age from 185. For example, if you are 40 years old your maximum heart rate would be 145. To determine your minimum training heart rate, simply subtract 20 from this number. In the case of a

40 year old this would be 125. So, the training zone would be a heartbeat between 125 and 145 beats per minute. For maximum health benefits you must stay in this range and never exceed it.

STEP 5 – DO IT OFTEN

You don't get in good physical condition by exercising once; it must be performed on a regular basis. A minimum of 15–20 minutes of exercising at your training heart rate at least three times a week is necessary to gain any significant cardiovascular benefits from exercise.

STEP 6 – MAKE IT FUN

The key to getting the maximum benefit from exercise is to make it enjoyable. Choose an activity that you enjoy and have fun with. If you can find enjoyment in exercise, you are much more likely to exercise regularly. One way to make it fun is to get a workout partner. For example, if you choose walking as your activity here is a great way to make it fun:

Find one or two people in your neighborhood that you would enjoy walking with. If you are meeting one or two people, you will certainly be more regular than if you depend solely on your own intentions. Commit to walking three to five mornings or afternoons each week, and gradually increase the exercise duration from an initial 10 minutes to at least 30 minutes.

STEP 7 – STAY MOTIVATED

No matter how committed a person is to regular exercise, at some point in time they are going to be faced with a loss of enthusiasm for working out. Here is a suggestion: take a break. Not a long break, just skip one or two workouts. It gives your enthusiasm and motivation a chance to recoup so that you can come back with an even stronger commitment. Here are some other things to help you to stay motivated:

SET EXERCISE GOALS. Being goal oriented helps keep us motivated. Success breeds success, so make a lot of small goals that can easily be achieved. Write down your daily exercise goal and check it off when you have it completed.

VARY YOUR ROUTINE. Variety is very important to help you stay interested in exercise. Doing the same thing every day becomes monotonous and drains motivation. Continually find new ways to enjoy working out.

KEEP A RECORD OF YOUR ACTIVITIES AND PROGRESS. Sometimes it is hard to see the progress you are making, but if you write in a journal you'll have a permanent record of your progress. Keeping track of your progress will motivate you to continue improving.

FINAL COMMENTS

When patients came to see me for help with stress, anxiety, or insomnia it amazed me how often they would say, "I don't have time to exercise." There is no question that many of these patients had extremely busy lives, but I just don't think that is a good enough excuse. You can always make time for exercise, whether it's getting up earlier, working out during lunch breaks, or sacrificing time spent on other activities. It's just too critical to avoid. The shorter your workout time, the greater the intensity of the workout must be.

CHAPTER 7

USE NATURAL PRODUCTS

The history of conventional medicine illustrates quite clearly how a treatment that is in vogue at a particular time can later be viewed as completely irrational and counter productive with the passage of time. Were the physicians of the late 19th century as convinced about the efficacy of the dominant treatments of the time (such as blood-letting and the use of toxic compounds, including mercury) as today's physicians are of their drug treatments? Undoubtedly, and sadly, the answer is yes. Certainly there are many safe and effective medical treatments, but I do believe there is a fundamental flaw in the use of most drugs. That flaw is that conventional drugs rarely produce a curative effect. Instead they simply act as biochemical band-aids to make us feel better.

In the relief of stress, anxiety, and insomnia this focus on symptom-relief often comes at a very high price. The drugs commonly prescribed are often highly addictive, create a dependency, interfere with normal physiology, and possess numerous side effects. Do not blindly be led into using drugs without first asking some important questions:

- What is the real benefit of taking this drug?

- What are the risks associated with either taking or not taking the drug?

- Are there any effective natural alternatives?

SEROTONIN

Before discussing natural products to use for stress, anxiety, and insomnia, it is important to mention that often people suffering from these conditions also suffer from depression, and vice-versa. This often reflects low levels of brain serotonin, an important neurotransmitter (a chemical messenger responsible for transmitting information from one nerve cell to another). Serotonin has been referred to as the brain's own mood-elevating and tranquilizing drug. There is a lot of support for this sentiment. Because the manufacture of serotonin in the brain is dependent upon how much tryptophan is delivered to the brain, in experimental studies researchers can remove tryptophan from the subject's diet and observe the effect it has. The results from these sorts of studies have contributed greatly to our understanding of just how vital proper levels of serotonin are to a positive human experience. Table 7.1 contrasts the different effects of optimal vs. low serotonin levels.

The lower the level of serotonin, the more severe the consequences. For example, low levels of serotonin are linked to depression with the lowest levels being observed in people who have committed or attempted suicide.

Table 7.1 – The Effects of Different Levels of Serotonin

OPTIMAL LEVEL OF SEROTONIN	LOW LEVEL OF SEROTONIN
Hopeful, optimistic	Depressed
Calm	Anxious
"Good-natured"	Irritable
Patient	Impatient
Reflective and thoughtful	Impulsive
Loving and caring	Abusive
Able to concentrate	Short attention span
Creative, focused	Blocked, scattered
Able to think things through	"Flies off the handle"
Responsive	Reactive
Does not overeat carbohydrates	Craves sweets and high carbohydrate foods
Sleeps well with good dream recall	Has insomnia and poor dream recall

ANTIDEPRESSANT DRUGS

In the treatment of depression conventional medicine primarily focuses on increasing the effects of serotonin. Once serotonin is manufactured in the brain it is stored in nerve cells waiting for release. Once released, the serotonin carries a chemical message by binding to receptor sites on the neighboring nerve cell. Almost as soon as the serotonin is released enzymes are at work that will either break down the serotonin or work to uptake the serotonin back into the brain cells. Either event terminates the serotonin effect. It is at this point that various drugs typically work, either inhibiting the reuptake of serotonin or preventing its breakdown. Most popular drugs of this type are referred to as SSRIs, short for Selective Serotonin Reuptake Inhibitors (see chart below). As a result of inhibiting serotonin reuptake, there is more serotonin hanging around capable of binding to receptor sites and transmitting the serotonin effect.

Table 7.2 – Examples of SSRIs

- Citalopram (Celexa, Cipramil, Cipram, Dalsan, Recital, Emocal, Sepram, Seropram, Citox, Cital)
- Dapoxetine (Priligy)
- Escitalopram (Lexapro, Cipralex, Seroplex, Esertia)
- Fluoxetine (Prozac, Fontex, Seromex, Seronil, Sarafem, Ladose, Motivest, Flutop)
- Fluvoxamine (Luvox, Fevarin, Faverin, Dumyrox, Favoxil, Movox)
- Paroxetine (Paxil, Seroxat, Sereupin, Aropax, Deroxat, Divarius, Rexetin, Xetanor, Paroxat, Loxamine, Deparoc)
- Sertraline (Zoloft, Lustral, Serlain, Asentra)
- Vilazodone (Viibryd)

The effectiveness of antidepressant drugs has been the subject of several reviews. The results indicate that they have not been shown to work any better than placebo in cases of mild to moderate depression (the most common reason for prescription medication), and claims that antidepressants are more effective in more severe conditions have little evidence to support them.[36, 37] In fact, the research indicates that SSRIs and other antidepressant drugs might actually increase the likelihood of suicides in adults and children.[38]

An additional alarming finding is that 25% of patients taking antidepressants do not even have depression or a diagnosable psychiatric problem.[39] So the bottom line is that millions of people are using antidepressants for a problem they do not have, and for the people who have a diagnosable condition, these medications do not work in most cases anyway and may cause significant side effects. As one group of researcher concluded, "Given doubt about their benefits and concern about their risks, current recommendations for prescribing antidepressants should be reconsidered."[36] This statement is a clear mandate to consider using natural medicine as a way to deal with the causes of these mood disorders.

While antidepressant drugs are at best only marginally successful in alleviating depression, they do produce many side effects. Approximately 20% of patients experience nausea; 20% headaches; 15% anxiety and nervousness; 14% insomnia; 12% drowsiness; 12% diarrhea; 9.5% dry mouth; 9% loss of appetite; 8% sweating and tremors; and 3% rashes. SSRIs also definitely inhibit sexual function. In studies where sexual side effects were thoroughly evaluated, 43% of men and women taking SSRIs reported loss of libido or diminished sexual response. There is also a significant risk for weight gain and the development of type 2 diabetes.

SSRIs, WEIGHT GAIN, AND DIABETES

A little-appreciated side effect of SSRIs is weight gain. Statistics show that once weight gain begins while taking these medications it usually does not stop. These drugs induce weight gain because they alter an area of the brain that regulates both serotonin levels and the utilization of glucose.[40] While the human brain usually makes up 2% of our overall body mass, it is so metabolically active that it uses up to 50% of the glucose in the body for energy. Evidently the SSRIs disrupt the utilization of glucose in the brain in such a way that the brain senses that it is low in glucose. That sets in motion very powerful signals to eat. And typically, if a person already has sugar cravings or other food urges, they will be dramatically enhanced by the drug. Other changes produced by the drug will lead to insulin resistance, setting the stage for inevitable weight gain and, perhaps, even type 2 diabetes. Studies have shown that individuals predisposed to diabetes are 2–3 times more likely to become diabetic if they use an antidepressant medication.[41]

ALTERNATIVES TO SSRIs

There are effective alternatives to antidepressant drugs. For example, there are a number of lifestyle and dietary factors that lead to reduced serotonin levels.

Chief among these factors are cigarette smoking, alcohol abuse, a high sugar intake, too much protein, blood sugar disturbances (hypoglycemia and diabetes), and various nutrient deficiencies. All of these factors have one thing in common – they lower serotonin levels by impairing the conversion of tryptophan to serotonin. A health-promoting lifestyle and diet go a long way towards restoring optimal serotonin levels and relieving depression. But, in the interim, natural agents like 5-HTP, S-adenosylmethionine (SAMe), or lavender extract can provide the boost in mood needed to help make important changes in diet and lifestyle easier to accomplish. Both natural agents are discussed below and a program for weaning off of SSRIs is given on page 84.

5-HYDROXYTRYPTOPHAN (5-HTP)

5-HTP is the direct building block for serotonin. It exerts significant advantages over L-tryptophan. While only 3% of an oral dose of L-tryptophan is converted to serotonin, more than 70% of an oral dose of 5-HTP is converted to serotonin. In addition to increasing serotonin levels, 5-HTP causes an increase in endorphin levels. Numerous double-blind studies have shown that 5-HTP is equal to SSRIs and tricyclic antidepressants in terms of effectiveness, but is less expensive, better tolerated, and associated with fewer and much milder side effects.[42, 43]

In many studies of depression, researchers use a rating scale called the Hamilton Depression Scale (HDS). The HDS score is determined by having the test subject complete a series of questions in which he or she rates the severity of symptoms on a numerical basis, as follows:

1 – present but mild   3 – severe

2 – moderate   4 – very severe

Symptoms assessed by the HDS include depression, feelings of guilt, insomnia, gastrointestinal symptoms, and other bodily symptoms of depression (e.g., headaches, muscle aches, heart palpitations), and anxiety. The HDS is popular in research because it provides a good assessment of the overall symptoms of depression. Table 7.3 shows the results of a study comparing 5-HTP to tryptophan and a placebo.

Table 7.3 – Hamilton Depression Scale from a comparative study of 5-HTP, Tryptophan, and Placebo

Result	5-HTP	Tryptophan	Placebo
Beginning of the study	26	25	23
End of the study (30 days)	9	15	19

In another study, 5-HTP was compared with the SSRI fluvoxamine (Luvox).[43] Fluvoxamine is used primarily in the United States as a treatment for obsessive compulsive disorder (OCD), an anxiety disorder characterized by obsessions and compulsions affecting an estimated 5 million Americans. Fluvoxamine exerts antidepressant activity comparable to (if not better than) other SSRIs like Prozac, Zoloft, and Paxil. In the study, subjects received either 5-HTP (100 mg) or fluvoxamine (50 mg) three times daily for six weeks. The assessment methods used to judge effectiveness included the HSD, the self-assessment depression scale (SADS), and physicians' assessments (Clinical Global Impression). As indicated in Table 7.4, the percentage decrease in depression was slightly better in the 5-HTP group (60.7% vs. 56.1%). The 5-HTP was quicker-acting than the fluvoxamine, and a higher percentage of patients responded to 5-HTP than to fluvoxamine.

Table 7.4 – Improvement in Specific Depression Symptoms

Symptom	5-HTP	Fluvoxamine
Depressed mood	67.5%	61.8%
Anxiety	58.2%	48.3%
Physical Symptoms	47.6%	37.8%

The advantages of 5-HTP over fluvoxamine were really evident when looking at the subcategories of the HDS: depressed mood, anxiety, physical symptoms, and insomnia, as shown in Table 7.4. However, perhaps more important than simply relieving insomnia is 5-HTP's ability to improve the quality of sleep. By contrast, antidepressant drugs greatly disrupt sleep processes.

The bottom line is that 5-HTP is equal to or better than standard antidepressant drugs, and the side effects are much less severe. In addition, many people prefer to use a natural substance like 5-HTP rather than synthetic drugs.

In the study comparing 5-HTP with fluvoxamine, here is how the physicians described the differences among the two groups: "Whereas the two treatment groups did not differ significantly in the number of patients experiencing side effects, the interaction between the degree of severity of the side effects and the type of medication was highly significant: fluvoxamine predominantly produced moderate to severe side effects, and 5-HTP produced primarily mild forms of side effects. Fourteen (38.9%) of the patients receiving 5-HTP reported side effects compared with 18 patients (54.5%) in the fluvoxamine group. The most common side effects with 5-HTP were nausea, heartburn, and gastrointestinal problems (flatulence, feelings of fullness, and rumbling sensations). These side effects were rated as being very mild to mild. In contrast, most of the side effects experienced in the fluvoxamine group were of moderate to severe intensity. The only subject to drop out of the 5-HTP group did so after five weeks, while four subjects in the fluvoxamine group dropped out after only two weeks. On the basis of studies on weight loss, the longer 5-HTP is used (e.g., after 4–6 weeks of use), the less the problem with mild nausea."

S-ADENOSYLMETHIONINE (SAMe)

Another alternative to SSRIs is SAMe, a compound that our bodies naturally produce, and which is involved in the manufacture of important brain chemicals including neurotransmitters and phospholipids like phosphatidylcholine and phosphatidylserine. Normally, the brain manufactures all the SAMe it needs from the amino acid methionine. However, SAMe synthesis is impaired in depressed patients. Supplementing the diet with SAMe in depressed patients results in increased levels of serotonin, dopamine, and phosphatidylserine, and improved binding of neurotransmitters to receptor sites, resulting in increased serotonin and dopamine activity, and improved brain cell membrane fluidity, and thus significant clinical improvement.[44]

The results of a number of clinical studies suggest that SAMe is one of the most effective natural antidepressants. Unfortunately, its use is still limited due to its high price, since many of the clinical trials used injectable SAMe. However, more recent studies using oral preparations have demonstrated that SAMe is just as effective orally as it is when given intravenously. SAMe is better tolerated, and gets results faster, than typical antidepressant drugs. Overall, in the double-blind studies comparing SAMe to antidepressant drugs, 76% of the SAMe group showed significant improvements in mood compared to only 61% in the drug group.[45, 46]

No significant side effects have been reported with oral SAMe. Generally the dosage for SAMe is 200 mg twice daily. If after two weeks no significant improvement is noted, the dosage can be increased to as much as 400 mg four times daily.

Individuals with bipolar disorder (manic depression) should not take SAMe. Because of SAMe's antidepressant activity, these individuals are susceptible to experiencing hypomania or mania (a state of heightened euphoria, mood, and/or energy) as it can aggravate the manic aspect of their condition. This effect is exclusive to some individuals with bipolar depression.

NUTRITIONAL PRODUCTS FOR STRESS AND ANXIETY

Two nutritional products useful for stress and anxiety in particular are L-theanine and GABA (specifically PharmaGABA).

CAFFEINE IN DEPRESSION AND ANXIETY

The importance of eliminating caffeine was stressed in Chapter 3 in regards to improving sleep quality. It also seems important in people prone to feeling depressed or anxious. Several studies have looked at caffeine intake and depression. For example, one study found that, among healthy college students, moderate and high coffee drinkers scored higher on a depression scale than did low users. Interestingly, the moderate and high coffee drinkers also tended to have significantly lower academic performance.[47] Several other studies have shown that depressed patients tend to consume fairly high amounts of caffeine (e.g., greater than 700 mg/day).[48, 49] In addition, caffeine intake has been positively correlated with the degree of mental illness in psychiatric patients.[50, 51]

The combination of caffeine and refined sugar seems to be even worse than either substance consumed alone. Several studies have found an association between this combination and depression. In one of the most interesting studies, 21 women and 2 men responded to an advertisement requesting volunteers "who feel depressed and don't know why, often feel tired even though they sleep a lot, are very moody, and generally seem to feel bad most of the time."[52] After baseline psychological testing, the subjects were placed on a caffeine- and sugar-free diet for one week. The subjects who reported substantial improvement were then given either a capsule containing caffeine and a Kool-Aid drink sweetened with sugar, or a placebo capsule containing cellulose and a Kool-Aid drink sweetened with an artificial sweetener, for up to six days. About 50% of the test subjects became depressed during the period where they were getting caffeine and sucrose.

Another study using a format similar to the Kool-Aid study found that 7 of 16 depressed patients were depressed during the caffeine and sugar challenge, but symptom-free while on the caffeine- and sugar-free diet and during the cellulose and artificial sweetener test period.[53]

The average American consumes 150–225 mg of caffeine daily, or roughly the amount of caffeine in 1–2 cups of coffee. Although most people appear to tolerate this amount, some people are more sensitive to the effects of caffeine than others. Even small amounts of caffeine, like what is found in decaffeinated coffee, are enough to affect some people adversely. The bottom line appears to be that anyone with depression or any psychological disorder should avoid caffeine completely.

L-THEANINE

L-theanine was discussed briefly in Chapter 3. It is a unique amino acid found almost exclusively in tea plants (*Camellia sinensis*). Clinical studies have demonstrated that L-theanine reduces stress, improves sleep quality, diminishes PMS symptoms, heightens mental acuity, and reduces the negative side effects of caffeine. These clinical effects are directly related to L-theanine's ability to stimulate the production of alpha brain waves (a state often achieved by meditation and characterized by being relaxed with greater mental focus and mental alertness) as well as reduce beta-waves (associated with nervousness, scattered thoughts, and hyperactivity).[21]

L-theanine has been approved for use in Japan as an aid to conquer stress and promote relaxation. It is a very popular ingredient in functional foods and beverages as well as dietary supplements designed to produce mental and physical relaxation without inducing drowsiness. L-theanine is fast acting. Generally, the effects are felt within the first 30 minutes, and have been shown to last up to 8–12 hours.

Based on the results of clinical studies, it has been established that L-theanine is effective in the range of 50–200 mg. If you have high levels of stress take at least 100–200 mg 1–3 times daily. Although L-theanine is completely safe and without any known adverse drug interaction, as a general guideline it is recommended to take no more than 600 mg within a six-hour period and no more than 1,200 mg within a 24-hour period.

PHARMAGABA

GABA (gamma-aminobutyric acid) is a natural calming agent found in the brain. In fact, it is one of the brain's most important neurotransmitters. It appears that many people with anxiety, insomnia, epilepsy, and other brain disorders do not manufacture sufficient levels of GABA. Many popular drugs such as Valium, Neurontin, baclofen, and Valproate act by increasing the effects of GABA within the brain.

PharmaGABA is a special form of GABA naturally manufactured from *Lactobacillus hilgardii* – the bacteria used to ferment vegetables in the preparation of the traditional Korean dish known as kimchi. Unlike chemically produced, synthetic GABA, PharmaGABA appears to be able to increase

WEANING OFF PRESCRIPTION DRUGS

If you are taking any prescription drug for stress, anxiety, depression, or insomnia and wish to discontinue, you need to work with your physician. In general, discontinuing any drug for these conditions has to be done gradually – especially with the benzodiazepines. The same is true for SSRIs. Stopping an SSRI too quickly is associated with symptoms such as dizziness, loss of coordination, fatigue, tingling, burning, blurred vision, insomnia, and vivid dreams. Less often, there may be nausea or diarrhea, flu-like symptoms, irritability, anxiety, and crying spells.

To provide support when weaning off of SSRIs, 5-HTP, and/or SAMe can be used. A concern when mixing antidepressant drugs with 5-HTP is producing what is referred to as the "serotonin syndrome" – characterized by confusion, fever, shivering, sweating, diarrhea, and muscle spasms. Although it is theoretically possible that combining 5-HTP with standard antidepressant drugs could produce this syndrome, to my knowledge no one has actually experienced this syndrome with the simultaneous use of 5-HTP and an SSRI. Nonetheless, my recommendation is that you be closely monitored by your doctor, when using 5-HTP in combination with standard antidepressant drugs, for any symptoms suggestive of the serotonin syndrome. If these symptoms appear, elimination of one of the SSRIs entirely may be indicated. There is no concern with using SAMe and SSRIs simultaneously.

Employing all of the general measures given in the previous chapters, reduce the dosage of the SSRI by 50% and take 50 mg of 5-HTP three times daily and/or 200 mg SAMe daily. After two weeks, reduce the dosage of the SSRI by half again. Stay on this dosage for a month before finally discontinuing the SSRI. If needed the dosage of 5-HTP can be increased to 100 mg three times daily and the dosage of SAMe can be as high as 400 mg four times daily.

brain alpha waves and lower beta waves. PharmaGABA is more powerful in this action than L-theanine, hence its effects are more noticeable.[54] Pharma-GABA has been shown to produce relaxation as evidenced by changes in brain wave patterns, pupil diameter, and heart rate, as well as to reduce other markers of stress including salivary cortisol levels. These effects are thought to be the result of activation of the parasympathetic nervous system rather than the PharmaGABA crossing the blood-brain barrier. Remember that activation of the parasympathetic nervous system produces the relaxation response.

Clinical studies with PharmaGABA have yielded some very interesting results. For example, one study had subjects who were afraid of heights walk across a long suspension bridge that spanned a 150-foot canyon. Halfway across the bridge a saliva sample was obtained and blood pressure was determined. What the researchers were looking for in the saliva was the level of secretory IgA – an important antibody in saliva that helps fight infection. During times of stress saliva levels of IgA typically drop, sometimes quite precipitously. This indeed happened when the subjects were given a placebo, but when they were given PharmaGABA the secretory IgA levels in the saliva were maintained halfway across the bridge and actually increased upon completion of the crossing.[54]

The typical dosage for PharmaGABA is 100–200 mg up to three times daily. Though no side effects have been reported, as a general guideline it is recommended to take no more than 1,000 mg within a 4-hour period and no more than 3,000 mg within a 24-hour period.

KEY BOTANICAL MEDICINES FOR STRESS

Several botanical medicines support adrenal function. Most notable are Chinese ginseng *(Panax ginseng)*, Siberian ginseng *(Eleutherococcus senticosus)*, rhodiola *(Rhodiola rosacea)*, and ashwagandha *(Withania somnifera)*. All of these plants exert beneficial effects on adrenal function and enhance resistance to stress, and are often referred to as "adaptogens" because they help us adapt to (cope with) stress. These plants have historically been used to:

- Restore vitality in debilitated and feeble individuals.

- Increase feelings of energy.

- Improve mental and physical performance.

- Prevent the negative effects of stress and enhance the body's response to stress.

In addition, I have found the water-soluble extract of lavender to be another important botanical that helps people cope with stress and anxiety. It works primarily to improve mood and promote a greater sense of serenity.

GINSENG

Both Siberian and Chinese ginseng have been shown to enhance our ability to cope with various stressors, both physical and mental.[55, 56] Presumably this anti-stress action is mediated by mechanisms that control the adrenal glands. Ginseng delays the onset and reduces the severity of the "alarm phase" of the body's short and long term response to stress (the general adaptation syndrome).

People taking either of the ginsengs typically report an increased sense of well-being. Clinical studies have confirmed that both Siberian and Chinese ginsengs significantly reduce feelings of stress and anxiety. For example, in one double-blind clinical study, nurses who had switched from day to night duty rated themselves for competence, mood, and general well-being, and were given a test for mental and physical performance along with blood cell counts and blood chemistry evaluation.[56] The group who were given Chinese ginseng demonstrated higher scores in competence, mood parameters, and mental and physical performance compared with those receiving placebos. The nurses taking the ginseng felt more alert, yet more tranquil, and were able to perform better than the nurses who were not taking the ginseng.

In addition to these human studies, animal studies have shown the ginsengs to exert significant anti-anxiety effects. In several of these studies, the stress-relieving effects were comparable to those of diazepam (Valium);

however, diazepam causes behavioral changes, sedative effects, and impaired motor activity, while ginseng has none of these negative effects.

On the basis of the clinical and animal studies, ginseng appears to offer significant benefit to people suffering from stress and anxiety. Chinese ginseng is generally regarded as being more potent than Siberian ginseng, and is probably better for the person who has experienced a great deal of stress, is recovering from a long-standing illness, or has taken cortico-steroids such as prednisone for a long time. For the person who is under mild to moderate stress and is experiencing less obvious impairment of adrenal function, Siberian ginseng may be the better choice. Dosages are as follows:

Chinese or Korean ginseng *(Panax ginseng):*

High-quality crude ginseng root: 1.5–2 g, 1–3 times daily

Fluid extract: 2–4 ml (½–1 tsp), 1–3 times daily

Dried powdered extract standardized to contain 5% ginsenosides: 250–500 mg, 1–3 times daily

Siberian ginseng *(Eleutherococcus senticosus):*

Dried root: 2–4 g, 1–3 times daily

Fluid extract (1:1): 2–4 ml (½–1 tsp), 1–3 times daily

Solid (dry powdered) extract (20:1 or standardized to contain more than 1% eleutheroside E): 100–200 mg, 1–3 times daily

RHODIOLA *(RHODIOLA ROSEA)*

Another useful botanical medicine to support stress management is *Rhodiola rosea* (arctic root), a popular plant in traditional medical systems in Eastern Europe and Asia, where it has traditionally been recommended to help combat fatigue and restore energy. Modern research has confirmed these effects and its adaptogenic qualities. However, the adaptogenic actions of rhodiola are different from those of the Chinese and Siberian ginsengs, which act primarily on the hypothalamus-pituitary-adrenal axis. Rhodiola seems to exert its adaptogenic effects by working on neurotransmitters and endorphins. It appears to offer an advantage over other adaptogens in circumstances of acute stress because it produces a greater feeling of relaxation and greater anti-anxiety effects. A single dose of rhodiola extract prior to acute stressful events has been shown to prevent stress-induced disruptions in function and performance, but like the ginsengs, it has also shown positive results with long-term use.[57-60] In one randomized, placebo-controlled trial of 60 patients with stress-related fatigue, rhodiola was found to have an anti-fatigue effect that increased mental performance, particularly the ability to concentrate, as well as decreasing the cortisol response to stress.[61]

On the basis of results of clinical trials with a standardized rhodiola extract, the therapeutic dose varies according to the rosavin content. For a dosage target of 3.6–7.2 mg of rosavin, the daily dose would be 360–600 mg for an extract standardized for 1% rosavin; 180–300 mg for 2% rosavin; and 100–200 mg for 3.6% rosavin. When rhodiola is used as an adaptogen, long-term administration is normally begun several weeks before the anticipated period of increased physiological, chemical, or biological strain, and continued throughout the duration of the challenging event or activity. When rhodiola is used as a single dose for acute stress (e.g., for an exam or an athletic competition), the suggested dose is three times the dose used for long-term supplementation. No side effects have been reported in clinical trials, but at higher dosages, some individuals might experience greater irritability and insomnia.

ASHWAGANDHA *(WITHANIA SOMNIFERA)*

A patented extract of roots and leaves from *Withania somnifera* know as Sensoril has shown impressive clinical results in dealing with stress. Developed by researcher Dr. S. Ghosal, Sensoril was the result of intense scientific investigations on the anti-stress action of various compounds in ashwagandha. Sensoril is standardized to contain the proper amounts of oligosaccharides, glycowithanolides, and Withaferin-A, that research has shown to promote optimal anti-stress activity.

Sensoril is derived from the freshly harvested roots and leaves of specially cultivated ashwagandha obtained from Northern regions of India. The roots used in Sensoril are from plants not more than two years old, as roots from older plants, which are used in many commercially available extracts of ashwagandha, may contain very little, if any, glycowithanolides.

Sensoril works with the body's natural biological systems to help restore balance to the body and normalize body functions. It helps to increase the body's resistance to stress and reduce physiological responses to stress events. Sensoril delivers a variety of benefits that help maintain good health.[62] Among other things, Sensoril:

- Helps counteract the negative effects of stress.
- Increases resistance to fatigue.
- Promotes mental clarity and concentration.
- Supports healthy weight management by inhibiting stress responses that can lead to overeating.
- Improves resistance to stress and tension.
- Helps protect against the effects of aging by protecting against free radical damage to cells.
- The typical dosage for Sensoril is 125 mg once or twice daily.

LAVENDER *(LAVANDULA OFFICINALIS)*

Lavender has long been used by herbalists as a treatment for anxiety, nervous exhaustion, and depression. Recently, this traditional treatment has been verified in a double-blind clinical trial.[63] The findings of the study indicated that taking a moderate amount of lavender can reduce feelings of depression, anxiety, and helplessness. In the study, 45 adults between the ages of 18 and 54 who were diagnosed with depression were assigned to one of three groups. The groups received either (1) lavender extract plus a placebo tablet, (2) a placebo plus 100 mg per day of the antidepressant drug imipramine, or (3) lavender extract and 100 mg per day of imipramine. The study lasted for four weeks and scores from the Hamilton Rating Scale for Depression (HAM-D, a questionnaire used to evaluate the severity of depression, where higher scores suggest more severe depression) were evaluated initially and then weekly after the start of treatment. What the results indicated was that the lavender extract was just as effective as the drug, but without the side effects common to drug treatment for depression (dry mouth, weight loss or weight gain, low blood pressure, arrhythmias, and decreased sexual function).

FINAL COMMENTS

The use of natural medicines as part of a stress management program can be tailored to your individual needs. Here is how I generally define the level of additional support that may be required:

LEVEL 1 SUPPORT

In addition to following the appropriate lifestyle and dietary approaches to stress reduction as well as regular utilization of techniques to calm the mind and body, Level 1 Support simply involves using natural products on an as-needed basis, such as following the recommendations in Chapter 3 for getting a good night's sleep (e.g., 5-HTP, L-theanine, and/or melatonin) or Chapter 4 for stabilizing blood sugar levels (PGX®), or taking L-theanine or PharmaGABA when experiencing situational stress.

LEVEL 2 SUPPORT

Level 2 Support involves all of the above and using either L-theanine or PharmaGABA on an ongoing basis due to more frequent feelings of stress or nervousness.

LEVEL 3 SUPPORT

Level 3 Support involves 1 and 2 above plus using one of the adrenal adaptogens on an ongoing basis, at the dosages recommended above.

LEVEL 4 SUPPORT

For people who are starting to experience or are experiencing significant signs of adrenal fatigue and generalized exhaustion, Level 4 Support is recommended. This level involves using all of the above plus a combination of the anti-stress botanicals. For example, two capsules of one formula I often recommend contain the following (the recommended dosage for Level 4 Support):

- Sensoril..250 mg
- Siberian ginseng extract..150 mg
  (standardized to contain 0.8% eleutherosides)
- Lavender extract (5:1)...150 mg
- Rhodiola extract..75 mg
  (standardized to contain 3.5% rosavins)

CONCLUSIONS

It is my sincere hope that in this book I have provided clear direction on steps that you can take to improve your life. The last few years I was in practice, it seemed that most of the patients I was seeing were seeking help with the very areas this book focuses on: stress, anxiety, insomnia, and depression. The changes that I witnessed in these patients after following my recommendations were truly astounding. One of the things that I noticed that appeared to be common to many of my patients was that before treatment they seemed to have lost the desire to engage in activities that would make them plugged into life. In short, they were not engaging in activities or interests that they used to be passionate about. They were often surprised that I spent a lot of time getting to know them on a personal level – their relationships, activities, day-to-day routine, stressors, etc. Often they left surprised, in that I had not only prescribed dietary advice, nutritional supplements, and herbal products, but also gave them what I felt might be a key "prescription" for helping them find passion in their lives again. On most occasions they would leave with this special prescription written out on a prescription pad, reminding them to breathe, and to engage in an activity they truly enjoyed. For one patient it might be taking his wife out to dinner or a movie. For another it might be visiting a friend they had not spoken to in months or years. For others it might be something as simple as enjoying a family night playing board games or having dinner with the neighbors. I found that if I could find something that would trigger the feelings that we all really need – love, friendship, appreciation, companionship, etc. – it made it much easier for me to help them feel good about their lives again.

So, I want to end this book by reminding you of that very important tool in changing your life – asking better questions. In Chapter 2 I stated that the quality of your life is equal to the quality of the questions you ask yourself. My all-time favorite question came to me one night when I was giving a speech to an audience of over 2,000 people at the Disneyland Hotel.

Like a lot of people, Disneyland holds a special place in my heart. My parents took me there when I was 12 years old. It was one of the highlights of my childhood – a very special memory. There's a reason why it's called the "Magical Kingdom." Twenty-six years later I was able to bring my parents with me when my wife and I took our daughter Lexi to Disneyland for her first time. To say the experience was overwhelming is putting it mildly. Holding my daughter when she spotted Mickey Mouse for the first time, while my wife and parents looked on, was one of the most magical moments of my life. I was holding pure joy and excitement in my very arms. Perhaps you have had a similar experience. I hope so. I cannot adequately express in words the feelings I experienced then and continue to experience every time I think about it.

Anyway, as I was finishing my speech to this group that night, I shared my Disneyland story and encouraged each of them to ask themselves the question, "How can I make my life more magical?" Almost as soon as I got the question out of my mouth, the answer occurred to me: *by making the lives of those around me more magical!* And I have found that applying the answer to that simple question has played a huge role in my life.

So, I want to end this book by asking you to ask yourself the same question: "How can I make my life more magical?" Think about it. Have fun thinking of how you can feel the magic by making a difference in someone else's life. Imagine how they will feel. And, then just go out and do it. To inspire you, let me share a quote that has been a great source of inspiration to me. It comes from the philosopher Goethe:

Until one is committed there is hesitancy, the chance to draw back, always ineffectiveness. Concerning all acts of initiative (and creation), there is one elementary truth, the ignorance of which kills countless ideas and splendid plans: that the moment one definitely commits oneself, then Providence moves too. All sorts of things occur to help one that would never have otherwise occurred. A whole stream of events issues from the decision, raising in one's favor all manner of unforeseen incidents and meetings and material assistance which no man could have dreamed would have come his way. Whatever you can do, or dream you can, begin it. Boldness has genius, power and magic in it. Begin it now!

Michael T. Murray, N.D.

APPENDICES

APPENDIX A – **THE STRESS SCALE**

The standard interpretation of the social readjustment rating scale is that a total of 200 or more units in one year is considered to be predictive of a high likelihood of experiencing a serious disease. However, rather than using the scale solely to predict the likelihood of serious disease, I recommend it as simply a tool to determine your level of exposure to stress, because everyone reacts differently to stressful events. If your score is greater than 200, however, I strongly encourage you to be very aggressive in your stress management.

Table A.1 The Social Readjustment Rating Scale[1]

Rank	Life event	Mean value
1	Death of spouse	100
2	Divorce	73
3	Marital separation	65
4	Jail term	63
5	Death of a close family member	63
6	Personal injury or illness	53
7	Marriage	50
8	Fired at work	47
9	Marital reconciliation	45
10	Retirement	45

11   Change in health of family member..44

12   Pregnancy..40

13   Sex difficulties...39

14   Gain of a new family member..39

15   Business adjustment...39

16   Change in financial state..38

17   Death of a close friend...37

18   Change to different line of work..36

19   Change in number of arguments with spouse............................35

20   Large mortgage...31

21   Foreclosure of mortgage or loan...30

22   Change in responsibilities at work...29

23   Son or daughter leaving home..29

24   Trouble with in-laws..29

25   Outstanding personal achievement..28

26   Spouse begins or stops work..26

27   Beginning or end of school...26

28   Change in living conditions...25

29   Revision of personal habits...24

30   Trouble with boss..23

31   Change in work hours or conditions...20

32   Change in residence..20

33   Change in schools...20

34   Change in recreation..19

35   Change in church activities...19

36   Change in social activities..18

37   Small mortgage...17

38   Change in sleeping habits...16

39   Change in number of family get-togethers..................................15

40   Change in eating habits..15

41   Vacation...13

42   Christmas...12

43   Minor violations of the law..11

APPENDIX B – **SELIGMAN'S ATTRIBUTIONAL STYLE QUESTIONNAIRE**

What distinguishes an optimist from a pessimist is the way in which they explain both good and bad events. Dr. Martin Seligman developed a simple test to determine your level of optimism (from *Learned Optimism*, Knopf, 1981). Take as much time as you need. There are no right or wrong answers. It is important that you take the test before you read the interpretation.

Read the description of each situation and vividly imagine it happening to you. Choose the response that most applies to you by circling either A or B. Ignore the letter and number codes for now; they will be explained after you take the test.

1. The project you are in charge of is a great success.	PsG
A I kept a close watch over everyone's work.	1
B Everyone devoted a lot of time and energy to it.	0
2. You and your spouse (boyfriend/girlfriend) make up after a fight.	PmG
A I forgave him/her.	0
B I'm usually forgiving.	1
3. You get lost driving to a friend's house.	PsB
A I missed a turn.	1
B My friend gave me bad directions.	0
4. Your spouse (boyfriend/girlfriend) surprises you with a gift.	PsG
A He/she just got a raise at work.	0
B I took him/her out to a special dinner the night before.	1
5. You forget your spouse's (boyfriend's/girlfriend's) birthday.	PmB
A I'm not good at remembering birthdays.	1
B I was preoccupied with other things.	0

6. You get a flower from a secret admirer.	PvG
A I am attractive to him/her.	0
B I am a popular person.	1
7. You run for a community office position and you win.	PvG
A I devote a lot of time and energy to campaigning.	0
B I work very hard at everything I do.	1
8. You miss an important engagement.	PvB
A Sometimes my memory fails me.	1
B I sometimes forget to check my appointment book.	0
9. You run for a community office position and you lose.	PsB
A I didn't campaign hard enough.	1
B The person who won knew more people.	0
10. You host a successful dinner.	PmG
A I was particularly charming that night.	0
B I am a good host.	1
11. You stop a crime by calling the police.	PsG
A A strange noise caught my attention.	0
B I was alert that day.	1
12. You were extremely healthy all year.	PsG
A Few people around me were sick, so I wasn't exposed.	0
B I made sure I ate well and got enough rest.	1
13. You owe the library ten dollars for an overdue book.	PmB
A When I am really involved in what I am reading, I often forget when it's due.	1
B I was so involved in writing the report that I forgot to return the book.	0
14. Your stocks make you a lot of money.	PmG
A My broker decided to take on something new.	0
B My broker is a top-notch investor.	1
15. You win an athletic contest.	PmG
A I was feeling unbeatable.	0
B I train hard.	1
16. You fail an important examination.	PsB
A I wasn't as smart as the other people taking the examination.	1
B I didn't prepare for it well.	0
17. You prepared a special meal for a friend and he/she barely touched the food.	PvB
A I wasn't a good cook.	1
B I made the meal in a rush.	0
18. You lose a sporting event for which you have been training for a long time.	PvB
A I'm not very athletic.	1
B I'm not good at that sport.	0

19. Your car runs out of gas on a dark street late at night.	PsB
A I didn't check to see how much gas was in the tank.	1
B The gas gauge was broken.	0
20. You lose your temper with a friend.	PmB
A He/she is always nagging me.	1
B He/she was in a hostile mood.	0
21. You are penalized for not returning your income tax forms on time.	PmB
A I always put off doing my taxes.	1
B I was lazy about getting my taxes done this year.	0
22. You ask a person out on a date and he/she says no.	PvB
A I was a wreck that day.	1
B I got tongue-tied when I asked him/her on the date.	0
23. A game show host picks you out of the audience to participate in the show.	PsG
A I was sitting in the right seat.	0
B I looked the most enthusiastic.	1
24. You are frequently asked to dance at a party.	PmG
A I am outgoing at parties.	1
B I was in perfect form that night.	0
25. You buy your spouse (boyfriend/girlfriend) a gift he/she doesn't like.	PsB
A I don't put enough thought into things like that.	1
B He/she has very picky tastes.	0
26. You do exceptionally well in a job interview.	PmG
A I felt extremely confident during the interview.	0
B I interview well.	1
27. You tell a joke and everyone laughs.	PsG
A The joke was funny.	0
B My timing was perfect.	1
28. Your boss gives you too little time to finish a project, but you get it finished anyway.	PvG
A I am good at my job.	0
B I am an efficient person.	1
29. You've been feeling run down lately.	PmB
A I never get a chance to relax.	1
B I was exceptionally busy this week.	0
30. You ask someone to dance and he/she says no.	PsB
A I am not a good enough dancer.	1
B He/she doesn't like to dance.	0

31. You save a person from choking to death.	PvG
A I know a technique to stop someone from choking.	0
B I know what to do in crisis situations.	1
32. Your romantic partner wants to cool things off for a while.	PvB
A I'm too self-centered.	1
B I don't spend enough time with him/her.	0
33. A friend says something that hurts your feelings.	PmB
A She always blurts things out without thinking of others.	1
B My friend was in a bad mood and took it out on me.	0
34. Your employer comes to you for advice.	PvG
A I am an expert in the area about which I was asked.	0
B I'm good at giving useful advice.	1
35. A friend thanks you for helping him/her get through a bad time.	PvG
A I enjoy helping him/her through tough times.	0
B I care about people.	1
36. You have a wonderful time at a party.	PsG
A Everyone was friendly.	0
B I was friendly.	1
37. Your doctor tells you that you are in good physical shape.	PvG
A I make sure I exercise frequently.	0
B I am very health-conscious.	1
38. Your spouse (boyfriend/girlfriend) takes you away for a romantic weekend.	PmG
A He/she needed to get away for a few days.	0
B He/she likes to explore new areas.	1
39. Your doctor tells you that you eat too much sugar.	PsB
A I don't pay much attention to my diet.	1
B You can't avoid sugar, it's in everything.	0
40. You are asked to head an important project.	PmG
A I just successfully completed a similar project.	0
B I am a good supervisor.	1
41. You and your spouse (boyfriend/girlfriend) have been fighting a great deal.	PsB
A I have been feeling cranky and pressured lately.	1
B He/she has been hostile lately.	0
42. You fall down a great deal while skiing.	PmB
A Skiing is difficult.	1
B The trails were icy.	0
43. You win a prestigious award.	PvG
A I solved an important problem.	0
B I was the best employee.	1

44. Your stocks are at an all-time low.	PvB
A I didn't know much about the business climate at the time.	1
B I made a poor choice of stocks.	0
45. You win the lottery.	PsG
A It was pure chance.	0
B I picked the right numbers.	1
46. You gain weight over the holidays, and you can't lose it.	PmB
A Diets don't work in the long run.	1
B The diet I tried didn't work.	0
47. You are in the hospital and few people come to visit.	PsB
A I'm irritable when I am sick.	1
B My friends are negligent about things like that.	0
48. They won't honor your credit card at a store.	PvB
A I sometimes overestimate how much money I have.	1
B I sometimes forget to pay my credit card bill.	0

Scoring Key

PmB: _____   PmG: _____

PvB: _____   PvG: _____

HoB: _____

PsB: _____   PsG: _____

Total B: _____   **Total G:** _____

G – B: _____

INTERPRETING YOUR TEST RESULTS

The test results will give you a clue as to your explanatory style. In other words, the results will tell you about how you explain things to yourself, or your habit of thought. Again, remember that there are no right or wrong answers.

There are three crucial dimensions to your explanatory style: permanence, pervasiveness, and personalization. Each dimension, plus a couple of others, will be evaluated on the basis of your answers to the questionnaire.

PERMANENCE

When pessimists are faced with challenges or bad events, they view them as being permanent. In contrast, people who are optimists tend to view the challenges or bad events as temporary. Here are some statements that reflect the subtle differences:

Permanent (Pessimistic)	Temporary (Optimistic)
"My boss is always a jerk."	"My boss is in a bad mood today."
"You never listen."	"You are not listening."
"This bad luck will never stop."	"My luck has got to turn."

To determine how you view bad events, look at the eight items coded PmB (for Permanent Bad): 5, 13, 20, 21, 29, 33, 42, and 46. Each answer with a "0" after it is optimistic; each one followed by a "1" is pessimistic. Total the numbers at the right-hand margin of the questions coded PmB, and write the total on the PmB line on the scoring key.

If you totaled 0 or 1, you are very optimistic on this dimension; 2 or 3 is a moderately optimistic score; 4 is average; 5 or 6 is quite pessimistic; and 7 or 8 is extremely pessimistic.

Now let us take a look at the difference in explanatory style between pessimists and optimists when there is a positive event in their lives. It is just the opposite of what happened with a bad event. Pessimists view positive events as temporary, whereas optimists view them as permanent. Here again are examples of some subtle differences in how pessimists and optimists might communicate their good fortune:

Temporary (Pessimistic)	Permanent (Optimistic)
"It's my lucky day."	"I am always lucky."
"My opponent was off today."	"I am getting better every day."
"I tried hard today."	"I always give my best."

Now total all the questions coded PmG (for Permanent Good): 2, 10, 14, 15, 24, 26, 38, and 40. Write the total on the line in the scoring key marked PmG.

If you totaled 7 or 8, you are very optimistic on this dimension; 6 is a moderately optimistic score; 4 or 5 is average; 3 is pessimistic; and 0, 1, or 2 is extremely pessimistic.

Are you starting to see a pattern? If you are scoring as a pessimist, you may want to learn how to be more optimistic. Your anxiety may be due to your belief that bad things are always going to happen and that good things are only "flukes."

PERVASIVENESS

Pervasiveness refers to the tendency to describe things either in universals (everyone, always, never, etc.) versus specifics (a specific individual, a specific time, etc.). Pessimists tend to describe things in universals, whereas optimists describe things in specifics, as shown in the following examples:

Universal (Pessimistic)	Specific (Optimistic)
"All lawyers are jerks."	"My attorney was a jerk."
"Instruction manuals are worthless."	"This instruction manual is worthless."
"He is repulsive."	"He is repulsive to me."

Total your score for the questions coded PvB (for Pervasive Bad): 8, 17, 18, 22, 32, 44, and 48. Write the total on the PvB line.

If you totaled 0 or 1, you are very optimistic on this dimension; 2 or 3 is a moderately optimistic score; 4 is average; 5 or 6 is quite pessimistic; and 7 or 8 is extremely pessimistic.

Now let us look at the level of pervasiveness of good events. Optimists tend to view good events as universal, and pessimists view them as specific. Again, it is just the opposite of how each views a bad event.

Total your score for the questions coded PvG (for Pervasive Good): 6, 7, 28, 31, 34, 35, 37, and 43. Write the total on the line labeled PvG.

If you totaled 7 or 8, you are very optimistic on this dimension; 6 is a moderately optimistic score; 4 or 5 is average; 3 is pessimistic; and 0, 1, or 2 is extremely pessimistic.

HOPE

Our level of hope or hopelessness is determined by our combined level of permanence and pervasiveness. Your level of hope may be the most significant score for this test. Take your PvB and add it to your PmB score. This is your hope score.

If it is 0, 1, or 2, you are extraordinarily hopeful; 3, 4, 5, or 6 is a moderately hopeful score; 7 or 8 is average; 9, 10, or 11 is moderately hopeless; and 12, 13, 14, 15, or 16 is severely hopeless.

People who make permanent and universal explanations for their troubles tend to have stress, anxiety, and depression; they tend to collapse when things go wrong. According to Dr. Seligman, no other score is as important as your hope score.

PERSONALIZATION

The final aspect of explanatory style is personalization. When bad things happen, we can either blame ourselves (internalize) and lower our self-esteem as a consequence, or we can blame things beyond our control (externalize). Although it may not be right to deny personal responsibility, people who tend to externalize blame in relation to bad events have higher self-esteem and are more optimistic.

Total your score for those questions coded PsB (for Personalization Bad): 3, 9, 16, 19, 25, 30, 39, 41, and 47.

A score of 0 or 1 indicates very high self-esteem and optimism; 2 or 3 indicates moderate self-esteem; 4 is average; 5 or 6 indicates moderately low self-esteem; and 7 or 8 indicates very low self-esteem.

Now let us take a look at personalization and good events; the pattern is the exact opposite of that for bad events. When good things happen, the person with high self-esteem internalizes, whereas the person with low self-esteem externalizes.

Total your score for those questions coded PsG (for Personalization Good): 1, 4, 11, 12, 23, 27, 36, and 45. Write your score on the line marked PsG on the scoring key.

If you totaled 7 or 8, you are very optimistic on this dimension; 6 is a moderately optimistic score; 4 or 5 is average; 3 is pessimistic; and 0, 1, or 2 is extremely pessimistic.

YOUR OVERALL SCORES

To compute your overall scores, first add the three B scores (PmB + PvB + PsB); the total is your B (bad event) score. Do the same for all of the G scores (PmG + PvG + PsG); the total is your G score. Subtract B from G to obtain your overall score.

If your B score is 3 to 6, you are marvelously optimistic when bad events occur; 10 or 11 is average; 12 to 14 is pessimistic; anything above 14 is extremely pessimistic.

If your G score is 19 or above, you think about good events extremely optimistically; 14 to 16 is average; 11 to 13 indicates pessimism; and a score of 10 or less indicates great pessimism.

If your overall score (G − B) is above 8, you are very optimistic across the board; if it is 6 to 8, you are moderately optimistic; 3 to 5 is average; 1 or 2 is pessimistic; and a score of 0 or less is very pessimistic.

APPENDIX C – **FREQUENTLY ASKED QUESTIONS ON PGX®**

WHAT IS PGX®?

PGX® (PolyGlycopleX®) is a unique complex of highly purified, water-soluble dietary fiber developed using advanced EnviroSimplex® technology. This technology combines these natural compounds in a very specific ratio making PGX® an effective weight loss aid and dietary supplement. PGX® was invented by researchers at InovoBiologic Inc., Calgary after many years of extensive research. PGX® is available in a variety of forms including capsules, soft gelatin capsules, granules, meal replacement powders, and pre-meal drink mixes.

WHERE CAN I BUY PGX®?

PGX® products are available under a variety of brand names, in stores throughout North America that sell natural health products. Visit pgx.com and select "Where to Buy" under the "About PGX®" main menu, enter an address, and click the "Find Nearest" button to see the nearest locations.

WHAT IS THE PGX® DAILY ULTRA MATRIX TECHNOLOGY?

PGX® technology has produced PGX® Daily Ultra Matrix Softgels – an advanced delivery system for optimum results. "Ultra Matrix" refers to PGX® granules suspended in a matrix of medium chain triglycerides (MCTs) – healthy fats from purified coconut oil. PGX® Daily disperses and becomes viscous slowly in the stomach and digestive tract. Most other fibers do not become as viscous as PGX®, become viscous too quickly, or do not become viscous at all. PGX® maintains its viscosity throughout the entire digestive tract (including the colon) which means that the glycemic index and subsequent blood sugar regulation is greater. Also, thanks to the thermogenic properties of the MCTs in the capsule, PGX® Daily can result in an extra 25–50 calories burned daily.

HOW DO I USE PGX®?

To enjoy the full benefits of PGX®, try to take some before each and every meal. Be sure to drink at least 250 ml (8 oz) of water per 2.5 gram serving of PGX®. Start with 1–2 softgels of PGX® Daily before each meal and increase by 1 softgel per meal every 2–3 days. If you are prone to digestive upset, increase the dose at a slower rate to give your body time to adjust. Some people find 2–3 softgels or 2.5 grams of PGX® granules to be effective. Others require the maximum dose of 6 softgels of PGX® Daily or 5 grams of PGX® granules in order to reduce portion size. Continue to increase the dosage until you experience a significant reduction in hunger and between-meal food cravings. Do not exceed 6 softgels or 5 grams up to three times per day.

DOES PGX® HAVE SIDE EFFECTS?

PGX® is a highly concentrated and highly effective form of fiber. It can take time for your body to adjust. To avoid minor side effects, such as increased gas, bloating, loose stools or constipation, it is best to start with small amounts of PGX® and then gradually increase your intake as your body adjusts. If you take PGX® consistently, and increase the dose gradually, it is likely that you will be able to consume a highly effective dose, without these effects, within a few days to a week. To decrease any possible side effects, it is important to drink a large glass of water with each dose of PGX®.

HOW FAST CAN I EXPECT TO LOSE WEIGHT?

Participants in a study who exercised and followed a 1,200 calorie/day diet lost on average 1–2 lbs per week. This is considered healthy weight loss. For some people weight loss is not immediate, while many people lose more weight depending upon their consistent use of PGX® and other lifestyle factors. PGX® makes following a calorie-restricted diet easy because it controls appetite due to its water solubility (absorbs many times its weight in water) and its ability to reduce and diminish cravings for starchy and sugary foods.

It is important to differentiate between weight loss and fat loss. As fat weighs less than muscle tissue, many people actually experience weight gain when they begin a reducing regime. Also, for some people, the additional water they drink with PGX® can temporarily add weight, since a liter of water weighs 1 kg or 2.2 lbs. While fast weight loss may seem ideal, it is important to remember that we gain weight gradually over a period of time. Losing weight the same way is "healthy weight loss" and will help reduce the risk of regaining the lost weight.

HOW DO I KNOW PGX® IS WORKING?
HOW MUCH DO I HAVE TO USE TO LOSE WEIGHT?

It is recommended that you start with a lower dose of PGX® for the first 3–7 days to see how your body adjusts to the increase in fiber intake. An increased amount of PGX®, to its active dosage (10–15 grams per day or 2.5–5 grams per meal) will produce noticeable reductions in appetite and cravings. Many people who have just started taking PGX® feel energized and notice their clothes fit better even though they have not changed anything else except taking PGX® everyday.

CAN PGX® BE TAKEN WITH MY MEDICATION?

PGX® can slow the rate of absorption of food and therefore it can theoretically do the same with medication. It is recommended that any oral medication be taken 1 hour before PGX® and/or 2–3 hours after consuming PGX® products. People with diabetes must monitor their blood glucose carefully as they may need to adjust medications accordingly. As PGX® helps control blood glucose, it may lessen the need for insulin or other medications over time. If you are on any medication consult a health care practitioner prior to using dietary supplements or changing your nutritional regimen.

CAN I TAKE PGX® WITH OTHER SUPPLEMENTS?

There is no problem taking PGX® along with supplements including essential fatty acids (EFAs) and multivitamins/multiminerals. A 21-day double-blind, placebo-controlled human tolerance study where 10 g of PGX® were given per day showed no statistical difference between levels of minerals and fat- and water-soluble vitamins in the test and control groups.

DOES PGX® CONTAIN GLUTEN?

PGX® softgels and PGX® granules are wheat and gluten free. PGX® meal replacement and pre-meal drink mix products cannot be considered gluten or wheat free.

IF PGX® IS FIBER HOW CAN I GET CONSTIPATED?

PGX® can only cause constipation if your water intake is not adequate for the amount of PGX® you are consuming. PGX® expands to hold many times its weight in water. You need to drink at least 250 ml (8 oz) of water per 2.5 grams (2–3 softgels). It is also important to eat smaller amounts of food regularly and take PGX® according to label directions. Be sure to take in adequate fresh water – not drinks such as coffee or alcohol that can cause you to lose water. During the day you may want to drink non-caffeinated herbal teas, vegetable juice, or diluted fruit juice (watch the sugar content of juices). Also, be sure to take PGX® consistently. Do not skip days and, if you are prone to constipation, take PGX® at the same time every day.

WHAT CAN I DO ABOUT GAS AND BLOATING?

Reduce the amount of PGX® you are taking and once you feel comfortable (no gas or bloating) gradually increase the amount over a few days (3–7 days). These side effects are temporary with most people and completely subside after a week or more of use. You may also want to take probiotic supplements (friendly intestinal bacteria) to enhance the health of your gastrointestinal tract.

AFTER TAKING PGX® IS IT POSSIBLE TO STILL BE HUNGRY?

For some people, yes. One explanation is that when blood sugar has been out of control or imbalanced for a long time, and the body has not been using insulin properly, the brain can still send out powerful messages to eat. When you take PGX® every day these strong messages become weaker. The inappropriate messages to eat are no longer needed when blood sugar becomes balanced and the brain is satisfied it will get the glucose required to function.

I'VE TRIED OTHER DIETS. HOW IS PGX® DIFFERENT?

PGX® isn't a diet, but it can make any weight loss plan or diet work better. Research has shown that people who gain weight and have difficulty losing weight, often spend much of their day on a "blood sugar roller coaster" with blood sugar alternately surging and plummeting, leaving them tired or irritable and leading to frequent and unhealthy food cravings. PGX® helps re-train your body and eliminate the blood sugar roller coaster so you don't crave "bad foods" and so you can better control your appetite. With PGX® you can achieve lasting results.

HOW DOES PGX® CONTROL CRAVINGS?

Often blood sugar levels can make our bodies crave sugar and starchy foods. Blood sugar levels rise and fall naturally, but rapid changes are harmful and create many of the cravings we experience. When blood sugar levels drop, our brain tells us to eat and often we look for foods with lots of sugars, fats, and starches in order to raise sugar levels. By balancing blood sugar levels, the brain is no longer demanding fast energy and you will be less likely to crave food.

DOES PGX® CONTAIN CAFFEINE OR OTHER STIMULANTS?

No. PGX® is a natural, non-addictive dietary supplement containing no caffeine or other stimulants.

HOW DO I KNOW IF MY BLOOD SUGAR IS "OUT OF BALANCE"?

Your doctor can do tests to determine whether or not your blood sugar levels are within normal range. The indicators you can see and feel yourself include:

- Cravings – especially sweets and carbohydrates.
- Feeling tired and irritable for no apparent reason.
- Gaining weight in spite of an unchanged diet or lifestyle.
- Feeling hungry again shortly after eating.

HOW DOES PGX® LOWER THE GLYCEMIC INDEX OF MEALS AND WHY IS THIS IMPORTANT?

Glycemic Index (GI) is a way of indicating how fast a particular food is turned into energy by the body. High GI foods are digested quickly and raise blood sugar fast. Low GI foods are converted to glucose more slowly. PGX® slows down the rate at which all food is digested, lowering after-meal blood sugar and virtually lowering the glycemic index of any food. Clinical studies show that high after-meal blood sugar levels are a major factor for heart disease risk.

HOW LONG DOES A PERSON HAVE TO TAKE PGX®?

After initial weight loss goals have been achieved, a lower "maintenance" dose of PGX® can effectively help control weight, appetite, blood sugar, and cholesterol for life. PGX® is non-habit forming but many people find that its effects – increased self esteem, a healthy weight, and more energy – are quite "addictive".

WHAT RESEARCH IS THERE TO SUPPORT THE BENEFITS AND EFFECTIVENESS OF PGX®?

PGX® is the result of many years of intensive clinical and laboratory research with universities from around the world and specialized research organizations in collaboration with the Canadian Centre for Functional Medicine. After years of research involving thousands of participants it is clear that adding PGX® to meals can: balance blood sugar, reduce the glycemic index of foods, restore insulin sensitivity (a key factor in weight control), curb food cravings, and lower cholesterol levels.

IS PGX® SUITABLE FOR CHILDREN?

Yes. Half the adult dose is recommended for children 9 years of age and older, or 1–3 softgels before each meal until the child notices a reduction in hunger and between-meal food cravings. However, children have unique developmental nutritional requirements. PGX® suppresses appetite and you should consult a qualified health care practitioner before giving PGX® to your child.

WHO SHOULD NOT USE PGX®?

Anyone who cannot compensate for a large water intake, such as someone with renal disease or congestive heart failure.

Anyone taking a large number of medications that must be taken with food and/or without food, unless advised by a health care practitioner.

Anyone who has difficulty swallowing, including people with gastrointestinal disorders and those with esophageal stenosis, or pre-existing bowel abnormalities, may be at risk for esophageal or intestinal blockages or obstruction and should consult a health care practitioner prior to use.

Pregnant or lactating women should discuss PGX® use with a health care practitioner prior to use.

Anyone under 18 years of age should discuss PGX® use with a health care practitioner prior to use.

If you have any concerns, consult a health care practitioner.

For more information on PGX® visit pgx.com

APPENDIX D – GLYCEMIC INDEX, CARBOHYDRATE CONTENT, AND GLYCEMIC LOAD OF SELECTED FOODS

A complete list of the glycemic index and glycemic load of all tested foods is beyond the scope of this book – it would be a book in itself. So I have selected the most common foods. This listing will give you a general sense of high GL and low GL foods. We have listed the items by food groups, from low to high glycemic loads. You may notice that certain food groups are not listed. For example, you won't see nuts, seeds, fish, poultry, and meats listed because these foods have little impact on blood sugar levels because they are low in carbohydrates.

If you would like to see an even more complete listing, visit mendosa.com – it's a free website operated by medical writer Rick Mendosa and an excellent resource.

FOOD	GI	Carbs g	Fiber g	GL
BEANS (LEGUMES)				
Soybeans, cooked, ½ cup, 100 g	14	12	7	1.6
Peas, green, fresh, frozen, boiled, ½ cup, 80 g	48	5	2	2
White navy beans, boiled, ½ cup, 90 g	38	11	6	4.2
Kidney beans, boiled, ½ cup, 90 g	27	18	7.3	4.8
Peas, split, yellow, boiled, ½ cup, 90 g	32	16	4.7	5.1
Lentils, ½ cup, 100 g	28	19	3.7	5.3
Lima beans, baby, ½ cup cooked, 85 g	32	17	4.5	5.4
Black beans, canned, ½ cup, 95 g	45	15	7	5.7
Pinto beans, canned, ½ cup, 95 g	45	13	6.7	5.8

FOOD	GI	Carbs g	Fiber g	GL
Chickpeas, canned, drained, ½ cup, 95 g	42	15	5	6.3
Kidney beans, canned and drained, ½ cup, 95 g	52	13	7.3	6.7
Broad, frozen, boiled, ½ cup, 80 g	79	9	6	7.1
Peas, dried, boiled, ½ cup, 70 g	22	4	4.7	8
Baked beans, canned in tomato sauce, ½ cup, 120 g	48	21	8.8	10
Blackeyed beans, soaked, boiled, ½ cup, 120 g	42	24	5	10
BREAD				
Multigrain, unsweetened, 1 slice, 30 g	43	9	1.4	4
Oat bran & honey, 1 slice, 40 g	31	14	1.5	4.5
Sourdough, rye, 1 slice, 30 g	48	12	0.4	6
Stoneground whole wheat, 1 slice, 30 g	53	11	1.4	6
Wonder, enriched white bread, 1 slice, 20 g	73	10	0.4	7
Sourdough, wheat, 1 slice, 30 g	54	14	0.4	7.5
Pumpernickel, 1 slice, 60 g	41	21	0.5	8.6
Whole wheat, 1 slice, 35 g	69	14	1.4	9.6
Healthy Choice, hearty 7-grain, 1 slice, 38 g	56	18	1.4	10
White (wheat flour), 1 slice, 30 g	70	15	0.4	10.5
Healthy Choice, 100% whole grain, 1 slice, 38 g	62	18	1.4	11
Gluten-free multigrain, 1 slice, 35 g	79	15	1.8	12
French baguette, 30 g	95	15	0.4	14
Hamburger bun, 1 prepacked bun, 50 g	61	24	0.5	15
Rye, 1 slice, 50 g	65	23	0.4	15
Light rye, 1 slice, 50 g	68	23	0.4	16
Dark rye, Black, 1 slice, 50 g	76	21	0.4	16
Croissant, 1, 50 g	67	27	0.2	18
Kaiser roll, 1 roll, 50 g	73	25	0.4	18
Pita, 1 piece, 65 g	57	38	0.4	22
Bagel, 1, 70 g	72	35	0.4	25
BREAKFAST CEREALS				
Oat bran, raw, 1 tablespoon, 10 g	55	7	1	4
Bran with psyllium, ⅓ cup, 30 g	47	12	12.5	5.6
Bran, ⅓ cup, 30 g	58	14	14	8
All-Bran Soy n Fiber, ½ cup, 45 g	33	26	7	8.5
All-Bran, ½ cup, 40 g	42	22	6.5.	9.2
Oatmeal (cooked with water), 1 cup, 245 g	42	24	1.6	10

FOOD	GI	Carbs g	Fiber g	GL
Shredded wheat, ⅓ cup, 25 g	67	18	1.2	12
Mini Wheats (whole wheat), 1 cup, 30 g	58	21	4.4	12
All-Bran Fruit n Oats, ½ cup, 45 g	39	33	6	13
Weet-Bix, 2 biscuits, 30 g	69	19	2	13
Cheerios, ½ cup, 30 g	74	20	2	15
Frosties, ¾ cup, 30 g	55	27	1	15
Corn Bran, ½ cup, 30 g	75	20	1	15
Honey Smacks, ¾ cup, 30 g	56	27	1	15
Wheatbites, 30 g	72	22	2	16
Total, 30 g	76	22	2	16.7
Healthwise for heart health, 45 g	48	35	2	16.8
Mini Wheats (blackcurrant), 1 cup, 30 g	71	24	2	17
Puffed wheat, 1 cup, 30 g	80	22	2	17.6
Bran Flakes, ¾ cup, 30 g	74	24	2	18
Crunchy Nut Cornflakes (Kellogg's), 30 g	72	25	2	18
Froot Loops, 1 cup, 30 g	69	27	1	18
Cocoa Pops, ¾ cup, 30 g	77	26	1	20
Team, 30 g	82	25	1	20.5
Corn Chex, 30 g	83	25	1	20.75
Just Right, ¾ cup, 30 g	60	36	2	21.6
Corn Flakes, 1 cup, 30 g	84	26	0.3	21.8
Rice Krispies, 1 cup, 30 g	82	27	0.3	22
Rice Chex, 1 cup, 30 g	89	25	1	22
Crispix, 30 g	87	26	1	22.6
Just Right Just Grains, 1 cup, 45 g	62	38	2	23.5
Oat n Honey Bake, 45 g	77	31	2	24
Raisin Bran, 1 cup, 45 g	73	35	4	25.5
Grape Nuts, ½ cup, 58 g	71	47	2	33.3
CAKE				
Cake, angel food, 1 slice, 30 g	67	17	<1	11.5
Cake, sponge cake, 1 slice, 60 g	46	32	<1	14.7
Cake, cupcake, with icing and cream filling, 1 cake, 38 g	73	26	<1	19
Cake, chocolate fudge, mix, (Betty Crocker), 73 g cake + 33 g frosting	38	54	<1	20.5
Cake, banana cake, 1 slice, 80 g	47	46	<1	21.6
Cake, pound cake, 1 slice, 80 g	54	42	<1	22.6

FOOD	GI	Carbs g	Fiber g	GL
Cake, French vanilla, (Betty Crocker), 73 g cake + 33 g frosting	42	58	<1	24.4
Cake, Lamingtons, 1, 50 g	87	29	<1	25
Cake, flan, 1 slice, 80 g	65	55	<1	35.75
Cake, scones, made from packet mix, 1 scone, 40 g	92	90	<1	83
CRACKERS				
Crackers, Corn Thins, puffed corn, 2, 12 g	87	9	<1	7.8
Crackers, Kavli, 4, 20 g	71	13	3	9.2
Crackers, Breton wheat crackers, 6, 25 g	67	14	2	9.4
Crackers, Ryvita or Wasa, 2, 20 g	69	16	3	11
Crackers, Stoned Wheat Thins, 5, 25 g	67	17	1	11.4
Crackers, Premium soda crackers, 3, 25 g	74	17	0	12.5
Crackers, water cracker, 5, 25 g	78	18	0	14
Crackers, graham 1, 30 g	74	22	1.4	16
Crackers, rice cake, 2, 25 g	82	21	0.4	17
MILK, SOY MILK, AND JUICES				
Milk, full fat, 1 cup, 250 ml	27	12	0	3
Soy, 1 cup, 250 ml	31	12	0	3.7
Milk, skim, 1 cup, 250 ml	32	13	0	4
Grapefruit juice, unsweetened, 1 cup, 250 ml	48	16	1	7.7
Nesquik chocolate powder, 3 tsp in 250 ml milk	55	14	0	7.7
Milk, chocolate flavored, low fat, 1 cup, 250 ml	34	23	0	7.8
Orange juice, 1 cup, 250 ml	46	21	1	9.7
Gatorade, 1 cup, 250 ml	78	15	0	11.7
Pineapple juice, unsweetened, canned, 250 ml	46	27	1	12.4
Apple juice, unsweetened, 1 cup, 250 ml	40	33	1	13.2
Cranberry juice cocktail (Ocean Spray USA), 240 ml	68	34	0	23
Coca Cola, 375 ml	63	40	0	25.2
Soft drinks, 375 ml	68	51	0	34.7
Milk, sweetened condensed, ½ cup, 160 g	61	90	0	55
FRUIT				
Cherries, 20 cherries, 80 g	22	10	2.4	2.2
Plums, 3–4 small, 100 g	39	7	2.2	2.7
Peach, fresh, 1 large, 110 g	42	7	1.9	3
Apricots, fresh, 3 medium, 100 g	57	7	1.9	4
Apricots, dried, 5–6 pieces, 30 g	31	13	2.2	4

FOOD	GI	Carbs g	Fiber g	GL
Kiwi 1 raw, peeled, 80 g	52	8	2.4	4
Orange, 1 medium, 130 g	44	10	2.6	4.4
Peach, canned, in natural juice, ½ cup, 125 g	38	12	1.5	4.5
Pear, canned, in pear juice, ½ cup, 125 g	43	13	1.5	5.5
Watermelon, 1 cup, 150 g	72	8	1	5.7
Pineapple, fresh, 2 slices, 125 g	66	10	2.8	6.6
Apple, 1 medium, 150 g	38	18	3.5	6.8
Grapes, green, 1 cup, 100 g	46	15	2.4	6.9
Apple, dried, 30 g	29	24	3.0	6.9
Prunes, pitted (Sunsweet), 6 prunes, 40 g	29	25	3.0	7.25
Pear, fresh, 1 medium, 150 g	38	21	3.1	8
Fruit cocktail, canned in natural juice, ½ cup, 125 g	55	15	1.5	8.25
Apricots, canned, light syrup, ½ cup, 125 g	64	13	1.5	8.3
Peach, canned, light syrup, ½ cup, 125 g	52	18	1.5	9.4
Mango, 1 small, 150 g	55	19	2.0	10.4
Figs, dried, tenderized (water added), 50 g	61	22	3.0	13.4
Sultanas, ¼ cup, 40 g	56	30	3.1	16.8
Banana, raw, 1 medium, 150 g	55	32	2.4	17.6
Raisins, ¼ cup, 40 g	64	28	3.1	18
Dates, dried, 5, 40 g	103	27	3.0	27.8
GRAINS				
Rice bran, extruded, 1 tbsp, 10 g	19	3	1	0.57
Barley, pearled, boiled, ½ cup, 80 g	25	17	6	4.25
Millet, cooked, ½ cup, 120 g	71	12	1	8.52
Bulgur, cooked, ⅔ cup, 120 g	48	22	3.5	10.6
Brown rice, steamed, 1 cup, 150 g	50	32	1	16
Couscous, cooked, ⅔ cup, 120 g	65	28	1	18
Rice, white, boiled, 1 cup, 150 g	72	36	0.2	26
Rice, Arborio risotto rice, white, boiled, 100 g	69	35	0.2	29
Rice, basmati, white, boiled, 1 cup, 180 g	58	50	0.2	29
Buckwheat, cooked, ½ cup, 80 g	54	57	3.5	30
Rice, instant, cooked, 1 cup, 180 g	87	38	0.2	33
Tapioca (steamed 1 hour), 100 g	70	54	<1	38
Tapioca (boiled with milk), 1 cup, 265 g	81	51	<1	41
Rice, jasmine, white, long grain, steamed, 1 cup, 180 g	109	39	0.2	42.5

FOOD	GI	Carbs g	Fiber g	GL
ICE CREAM				
Ice cream, low-fat French vanilla, 100 ml	38	15	0	5.7
Ice cream, full fat, 2 scoops, 50 g	61	10	0	6.1
JAM				
Jam, no sugar, 1 tbsp, 25 g	55	11	<1	6
Jam, sweetened 1 tbsp	48	17	<1	8
MUFFINS AND PANCAKES				
Muffins, chocolate butterscotch, from mix, 50 g	53	28	1	15
Muffins, apple, oat and sultana, from mix, 50 g	54	28	1	15
Muffins, apricot, coconut and honey, from mix, 50 g	60	27	1.5	16
Muffins, banana, oat and honey, from mix, 50 g	65	28	1.5	18
Muffins, apple, 1 muffin, 80 g	44	44	1,5	19
Muffins, bran, 1 muffin, 80 g	60	34	2.5	20
Muffins, blueberry, 1 muffin, 80 g	59	41	1,5	24
Pancake, buckwheat, from dry mix, 40 g	102	30	2	30
Pancake, from dry mix, 1 large, 80 g	67	58	1	39
PASTA				
Pasta, tortellini, cheese, cooked, 180 g	50	21	2	10.5
Pasta, ravioli, meat-filled, cooked, 1 cup, 220 g	39	30	2	11.7
Pasta, vermicelli, cooked, 1 cup, 180 g	35	45	2	15.7
Pasta, rice noodles, fresh, boiled, 1 cup, 176 g	40	44	0.4	17.6
Pasta, spaghetti, whole meal, cooked, 1 cup, 180 g	37	48	3.5	17.75
Pasta, fettuccine, cooked, 1 cup, 180 g	32	57	2	18.2
Pasta, spaghetti, gluten free, in tomato sauce, 1 small tin, 220 g	68	27	2	18.5
Pasta, macaroni and cheese, packaged, cooked, 220 g	64	30	2	19.2
Pasta, Star Pastina, cooked, 1 cup, 180 g	38	56	2	21
Pasta, spaghetti, white, cooked, 1 cup, 180 g	41	56	2	23
Pasta, rice pasta, brown, cooked, 1 cup, 180 g	92	57	2	52
SUGARS				
Fructose, 10 g	23	10	0	2.3
Honey, ½ tablespoon, 10 g	58	16	0	4.6
Lactose, 10 g	46	10	0	4.6
Sucrose, 10 g	65	10	0	6.5
Glucose, 10 g	102	10	0	10.2
Maltose, 10 g	105	10	0	10.5

FOOD	GI	Carbs g	Fiber g	GL
SNACKS				
Corn chips, Doritos original, 50 g	42	33	<1	13.9
Snickers, 59 g	41	35	0	14.3
Tofu frozen dessert (non-dairy), 100 g	115	13	<1	15
Real Fruit bars, strawberry, 20 g	90	17	<1	15.3
Twix cookie bar (caramel), 59 g	44	37	<1	16.2
Pretzels, 50 g	83	22	<1	18.3
Mars bar, 60 g	65	41	0	26.6
Skittles, 62 g	70	55	0	38.5
SOUPS				
Tomato, canned, 220 ml	38	15	1.5	6
Black bean, 220 ml	64	9	3.4	6
Lentil, canned, 220 ml	44	14	3	6
Split pea, canned, 220 ml	60	13	3	8
VEGETABLES				
Carrots, raw, ½ cup, 80 g	16	6	1.5	1
Carrots, peeled, boiled, ½ cup, 70 g	49	3	1.5	1.5
Beets, canned, drained, 2–3 slices, 60 g	64	5	1	3
Pumpkin, peeled, boiled, ½ cup, 85 g	75	6	3.4	4.5
Parsnips, boiled, ½ cup, 75 g	97	8	3	8
Sweet corn on the cob, boiled 20 min, 80 g	48	14	2.9	8
Corn, canned and drained, ½ cup, 80 g	55	15	3	8.5
Sweet potato, peeled, boiled, 80 g	54	16	3.4	8.6
Sweet corn, ½ cup boiled, 80 g	55	18	3	10
Potatoes, peeled, boiled, 1 medium, 120 g	87	13	1.4	10
Potatoes, with skin, boiled, 1 medium, 120 g	79	15	2.4	11
Yam, boiled, 80 g	51	26	3.4	13
Potatoes, baked in oven (no fat), 1 medium, 120 g	93	15	2.4	14
Potatoes, mashed, ½ cup, 120 g	91	16	1	14
Potatoes, Instant potato, prepared, ½ cup	83	18	1	15
Potatoes, new, unpeeled, boiled, 5 small (cocktail), 175 g	78	25	2	20
Cornmeal (polenta), ⅓ cup, 40 g	68	30	2	20
Potatoes, French fries, fine cut, small serving, 120 g	75	49	1	36
Gnocchi, cooked, 1 cup, 145 g	68	71	1	48

FOOD	GI	Carbs g	Fiber g	GL
LOW GLYCEMIC VEGETABLES				
Asparagus, 1 cup, cooked or raw Bell Peppers, 1 cup, cooked or raw Broccoli, 1 cup, cooked or raw Brussels sprouts, 1 cup, cooked or raw Cabbage, 1 cup, cooked or raw Cauliflower, 1 cup, cooked or raw Cucumber, 1 cup Celery, 1 cup, cooked or raw Eggplant, 1 cup Green beans, 1 cup, cooked or raw Kale, 1 cup cooked, 2 cups raw Lettuce, 2 cups raw Mushrooms, 1 cup Spinach, 1 cup cooked, 2 cups raw Tomatoes, 1 cup Zucchini, 1 cup, cooked or raw	≈20	≈7	≈1.5	≈1.4
YOGURT				
Yogurt, low fat, artificial sweetener, 200 g	14	12	0	2
Yogurt, with fruit, 200 g	26	30	0	8
Yogurt, low fat, 200 g	33	26	0	8.5

APPENDIX E – THE OPTIMAL HEALTH FOOD PYRAMID

The Optimal Health Food Pyramid, shown below, incorporates the best from two of the most healthful diets ever studied – the traditional Mediterranean diet and the traditional Asian diet. In addition, the Optimal Health Food Pyramid more clearly defines what the healthy components within the categories are and stresses the importance of vegetable oils and regular fish consumption as part of a healthful diet.

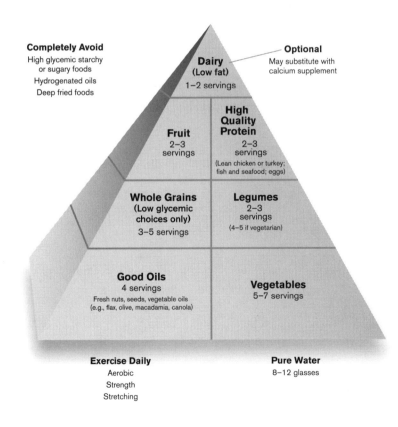

Completely Avoid
High glycemic starchy or sugary foods
Hydrogenated oils
Deep fried foods

Optional
May substitute with calcium supplement

Dairy
(Low fat)
1–2 servings

High Quality Protein
2–3 servings
(Lean chicken or turkey; fish and seafood; eggs)

Fruit
2–3 servings

Whole Grains
(Low glycemic choices only)
3–5 servings

Legumes
2–3 servings
(4–5 if vegetarian)

Good Oils
4 servings
Fresh nuts, seeds, vegetable oils
(e.g., flax, olive, macadamia, canola)

Vegetables
5–7 servings

Exercise Daily
Aerobic
Strength
Stretching

Pure Water
8–12 glasses

FOODS TO AVOID ENTIRELY

- Refined white flour products: pastas, cakes, muffins, pretzels, etc.

- Refined sugar-loaded cereals, candies, baked goods, etc.

- Processed foods packed full of empty calories (sugar and fat) or salt (e.g., soups, theater-style popcorn, chips, etc.)

- Margarine, butter, and shortening

- Smoked or cured meats: bacon, hot dogs, smoked luncheon meats, sausages, ham, spam, etc.

- Meats cooked at extremely high temperatures or cooked to well done

- Heavily sweetened or artificially sweetened soft drinks, Kool-Aid, juice-flavored drinks, etc.

- Fried foods, including French fries, potato chips, corn chips, and doughnuts

Table E.1 Daily food group recommendations for a 2,000-calorie diet

FOOD	NO. SERVINGS
Vegetables	
Total servings	5–7
Green leafy and cruciferous vegetables	2–4
Low-glycemic vegetables	2–3
Other vegetables	1–2
Good Oils	
Total servings	4
Nuts and seeds	1
Olive, macadamia, flaxseed, or canola oil	2–3
Whole Grains	3–5
Legumes	2–3 (4–5 if vegetarian)
High-Quality Protein	2–3
Fruit	2–3
Dairy	1–2 (optional)

VEGETABLES: FIVE TO SEVEN SERVINGS DAILY

In Latin, the word vegetable means "to enliven or animate." Vegetables give us life and should be the main focus of any health-promoting diet. Vegetables provide the broadest range of nutrients of any food class. They are rich sources of vitamins, minerals, carbohydrates, and protein. Vegetables also provide high quantities of anticancer phytochemicals.

It is very important not to overcook vegetables. Overcooking not only results in loss of important nutrients, but it also alters the flavor of the vegetable. Light steaming, baking, and quick stir frying are the best ways to cook vegetables. Do not boil vegetables unless you are making soup, as much of the nutrients will leach into the water. If fresh vegetables are not available, frozen vegetables are preferred over their canned counterparts. The only exception is tomato products (e.g., soup, paste, sauce, etc.), especially when they also contain oil; canned tomato products actually provide more absorbable lycopene than raw tomatoes.

We have divided vegetable intake into three categories: green leafy and cruciferous vegetables; low-glycemic vegetables; and starchy vegetables. This approach encourages eating a variety of these life-giving foods, helps achieve a "rainbow assortment" in the diet, and enables a focus on low-glycemic choices.

One serving of vegetables equals any of the following:

- 1 cup raw leafy vegetables (such as lettuce or spinach)
- ½ cup raw non-leafy vegetables
- ½ cup cooked vegetables or fresh vegetable juice

Green Leafy and Cruciferous Vegetables: Two to Four Servings Daily

Alfalfa sprouts	Beet greens	Bok choy
Broccoli	Brussels sprouts	Cabbage
Cauliflower	Chard	Chinese cabbage
Collard greens	Dandelion	Endive

Escarole	Kale	Lettuce (the darker,
Mustard greens	Parsley	the better)
Spinach	Turnip greens	Watercress

Low-Glycemic Vegetables: Two to Three Servings Daily

Artichoke (one medium)	Asparagus	Bean sprouts
Bell peppers	Carrots	Celery
Cucumber	Fennel	Mushrooms
Okra	Onions	Peas (fresh or frozen)
Radishes	Rhubarb	String beans, green or
Summer squash	Tomatoes, tomato paste,	yellow
Zucchini	tomato sauce, tomato	
	juice, vegetable juice cocktail	

Starchy Vegetables: One to Two Servings Daily

Beets	Parsnip	Potato
Pumpkin	Rhubarb	Rutabaga
Winter, acorn, or	Yam or sweet potato	
butternut squash		

NUTS, SEEDS, AND GOOD OILS: FOUR SERVINGS DAILY

Nuts and seeds provide the beneficial oils, especially the monounsaturated and medium-chain fatty acids. Regular consumption of nuts has been shown to improve blood sugar regulation and lower the risk for diabetes, heart disease, obesity, and cancer. Focus on raw nuts and seeds. Definitely avoid nuts and seeds roasted in oils or coated with sugar. Nuts and seeds make excellent additions to salads and sautéed greens. Try to eat a variety of nuts and seeds, such as almonds, Brazil nuts, walnuts, pecans, flaxseeds, sunflower seeds, and pumpkin seeds.

Use olive, macadamia, flaxseed, or canola oil both in salad dressings and to replace butter, margarine, and shortening used for cooking. Never cook with flaxseed oil; it is too rich in polyunsaturated fats, which are easily damaged by heat. Coconut and macadamia nut oil are the best cooking oils because of their ability to remain stable during high temperatures, but olive oil is a good choice for sautéed vegetables, and canola oil is usually best for baked goods because it has the mildest flavor. Coconut oil is also very stable in cooking and is fine to use in small quantities; it contains saturated fat but is metabolized differently from animal-derived saturated fats and can be used safely in moderation. Avoid using safflower, sunflower, soy, and corn oils because they contain too much omega-6 fatty acid.

We recommend at least one serving of nuts or seeds (one serving equals ¼ cup) and 3 tbsp of the healthy oils daily. In addition, we recommend taking a high-quality fish oil supplement.

WHOLE GRAINS: THREE TO FIVE SERVINGS DAILY

It is very important to choose whole-grain products (e.g., whole-grain breads, whole-grain flour products, brown rice) over their processed counterparts (white bread, white flour products, white rice, etc.). Whole grains provide substantially more nutrients and health-promoting properties. Whole grains are a major source of complex carbohydrates, dietary fiber, magnesium and other minerals, and B vitamins. The content and quality of the protein in whole grains are also greater than in refined grains. Diets rich in whole grains have been shown to be helpful in both prevention and treatment of diabetes, heart disease, and cancer.

Table E.2 Single servings of whole grains

FOOD	SINGLE SERVING
Bread	
Whole wheat, rye, or other whole grain	1 slice
Cereals	
Whole grain	½ cup
Corn	
Cooked whole kernel corn	½ cup
Corn on the cob	1 small

Flour and Flour Products	
Whole-wheat flour (uncooked)	2½ tbsp
Whole-grain pasta (cooked)	½ cup
Whole grains (cooked): rice, oats, wheat, barley, quinoa, spelt, etc.	½ cup

BEANS (LEGUMES): TWO TO THREE SERVINGS DAILY

Beans are a mainstay in most diets of the world and are second only to grains in supplying calories and protein to the world's population. Compared with grains, they supply about the same number of total calories, but usually provide two to four times as much protein, and are a richer source of the soluble fiber that lowers cholesterol and stabilizes blood glucose levels. Although we do not recommend using canned vegetables or fruit, canned beans retain their fiber content and anticancer flavonoids. Plus, given the long preparation time for cooking beans, canned beans are extremely quick and convenient.

A serving size for beans is ½ cup.

FRUITS: THREE TO FOUR SERVINGS DAILY

Fruits are a rich source of many beneficial nutrients, and regular fruit consumption has been shown to offer significant protection against chronic degenerative diseases, including cancer, heart disease, cataracts, diabetes, and strokes. Fruits make nutrient dense, easy between meal snacks and desserts (e.g., nothing could be simpler than phytonutrient-rich fresh berries alone). It is easy to get into the habit of eating only a few varieties of fruit. We encourage eating a "rainbow assortment" of fruits over the course of a week.

A general rule of thumb is that one serving of fruit equals one of the following:

- One medium fruit
- ½ cup of small or cut-up fruit

- 4 oz of 100% juice
- ¼ cup dried fruit

HIGH-QUALITY PROTEIN: TWO TO THREE SERVINGS DAILY

The detriment of diets high in saturated fat and cholesterol has been stressed for decades. Likewise, the importance of the omega-3 fatty acids in the battle against development of chronic disease is now also well known. Fish consumption, in particular, has shown tremendous protection against heart disease and cancer. Choose smaller species of fatty fish, such as wild salmon, mackerel, herring, and sardines. Their smaller size and shorter lifespan translate into a lower accumulation of mercury.

I recommend eating fish at least three, but no more than six, times per week. Keep intake of red meat (beef, veal, or lamb) to no more than two servings per month, and choose the leanest cuts possible; keep the portion size limited to about the size of a deck of cards, and do not charbroil or cook the meat until well done, because this practice increases the formation of cancer-causing compounds. Also, consider some of the alternatives to beef, such as venison, buffalo, elk, rabbit, and ostrich; these emerging beef alternatives are lower in saturated fat and provide higher levels of omega-3 fatty acids.

Chicken and turkey can also provide excellent protein with very little fat, especially if only the white meat (breast) without the skin is eaten. Eggs are also a very good source of high-quality protein, and if produced by free-range hens fed flaxseed meal, they will be rich in beneficial omega-3 fatty acids.

One serving equals about the size of a deck of cards; that translates to roughly 4 oz.

DAIRY: ONE OR TWO SERVINGS DAILY (OPTIONAL)

We have found that many people are allergic to milk or lack the enzymes necessary to digest dairy products. Even for people who do tolerate dairy foods, milk consumption should be limited to no more than one or two servings per day. Use nonfat or reduced fat dairy products rather than whole milk varieties. Also, fermented dairy products like yogurt, kefir, and acidophilus-fortified milk are preferred over milk. Some of the soy milk alternatives to cow's milk are delicious, especially when flavored with vanilla or chocolate. If dairy products are not consumed, we recommend a calcium supplement.

One serving of dairy products equals 1 cup of milk, yogurt, or cottage cheese or 1 oz of cheese.

REFERENCES

The references provided are by no means designed to represent a complete reference list for all of the studies reviewed or mentioned in this book. In fact, I have chosen to focus on key studies and comprehensive review articles that readers, especially medical professionals, may find helpful.

If you are interested in reading the studies cited or wish more information on additional studies, visit the website for the National Library of Medicine (NLM) at http://gateway.nlm.nih.gov. The NLM Gateway is a web-based system that lets users search simultaneously in multiple retrieval systems at the NLM. From this site you can access all of the NLM databases, including the PubMed database. The PubMed database was developed in conjunction with publishers of biomedical literature as a search tool for accessing literature citations and linking to full-text journal articles at websites of participating publishers. Publishers participating in PubMed electronically supply NLM with their citations prior to or at the time of publication. If the publisher has a website that offers full text of its journals, PubMed provides links to that site, as well as sites with other biological data, sequence centers, etc. User registration, a subscription fee, or some other type of fee may be required to access the full text of articles in some journals.

PubMed provides access to bibliographic information, including MEDLINE – the NLM's premier bibliographic database covering the fields of medicine, nursing, dentistry, veterinary medicine, the health care system, and the preclinical sciences. MEDLINE contains bibliographic citations and author abstracts from more than 4,000 medical journals published in the United States and 70 other countries. The file contains over 12 million citations dating back to the mid-1960s. Coverage is worldwide, but most records are from English-language sources or have English abstracts (summaries). Conducting a search is quite easy and the site has a link to a tutorial that fully explains the search process.

REFERENCES

1   Holmes TH, Rahe RH. The social readjustment rating scale. *J Psychosom Res*. 1967; 11:213-218.

2   Törnhage CJ. Salivary cortisol for assessment of hypothalamic-pituitary-adrenal axis function. *Neuroimmunomodulation*. 2009; 16(5):284-9.

3   Lewis JG. Steroid Analysis in Saliva: An overview. *Clin Biochem Rev*. 2006 Aug; 27(3):139-46.

4   Stetler C, Miller GE. Blunted cortisol response to awakening in mild to moderate depression: regulatory influences of sleep patterns and social contacts. *J Abnorm Psychol*. 2005 Nov; 114(4):697-705.

5   Backhaus J, Junghanns K, Hohagen F. Sleep disturbances are correlated with decreased morning awakening salivary cortisol. *Psychoneuroendocrinology*. 2004 Oct; 29(9):1184-91.

6   Benson H. *The relaxation response*. New York: William Morrow, 1975.

7   Kripke DF. Chronic hypnotic use: deadly risks, doubtful benefit. *Sleep Med Rev*. 2000 Feb; 4(1):5-20.

8   Mallon L, Broman JE, Hetta J. Is usage of hypnotics associated with mortality? *Sleep Med*. 2009 Mar; 10(3):279-86.

9   Kripke DF. Do hypnotics cause death and cancer? The burden of proof. *Sleep Med*. 2009 Mar; 10(3):275-6.

10 Kripke DF. Possibility that certain hypnotics might cause cancer in skin. *J Sleep Res*. 2008 Sep; 17(3):245-50.

11 Olde Rikkert MG, Rigaud AS. Melatonin in elderly patients with insomnia. A systematic review. *Z Gerontol Geriatr*. 2001; 34:491-497.

12 Haimov I, Lavie P, Laudon M, *et al*. Melatonin replacement therapy of elderly insomniacs. *Sleep*. 1995; 18:598-603.

13   Dollins AB, Zhdanova IV, Wurtman RJ, *et al.* Effect of inducing nocturnal serum melatonin concentrations in daytime on sleep, mood, body temperature, and performance. *Proc Natl Acad Sci.* USA 1994; 91:1824-1828.

14   Mallo C, Zaidan R, Faure A, *et al.* Effects of a four-day nocturnal melatonin treatment on the 24 h plasma melatonin, cortisol and prolactin profiles in humans. *Acta Endocrinol.* (Copenh) 1988; 119:474-480.

15   Wyatt RJ. The serotonin-catecholamine-dream bicycle. A clinical study. *Biol Psychiatry.* 1972; 5:33-64.

16   Guilleminault C, Cathala HP, Castaigne P. Effects of 5-HTP on sleep of a patient with brain stem lesion. *Electroencephalogr Clin Neurophysiol.* 1973; 34:177-184.

17   Wyatt RJ, Zarcone V, Engelman K. Effects of 5-hydroxytryptophan on the sleep of normal human subjects. *Electroencephalogr Clin Neurophysiol.* 1971; 30:505-509.

18   Autret A, Minz M, Bussel B, *et al.* Human sleep and 5-HTP. Effects of repeated high doses and of association with benserazide. *Electroencephalogr Clin Neurophysiol.* 1976; 41:408-413.

19   Zarcone VP Jr, Hoddes E. Effects of 5-hydroxytryptophan on fragmentation of REM sleep in alcoholics. *Am J Psychiatry.* 1975; 132:74-76.

20   Soulairac A, Lambinet H. Effect of 5-hydroxytryptophan, a serotonin precursor, on sleep disorders. *Ann Med Psychol.* (Paris) 1977; 1:792-798.

21   Eschenauer G, Sweet BV. Pharmacology and therapeutic uses of theanine. *Am J Health Syst Pharm.* 2006; 63(1):26, 28-30.

22   Stevinson C, Ernst E. Valerian for insomnia: a systematic review of randomized clinical trials. *Sleep Med.* 2000; 1:91-99.

23   Hadley S, Petry JJ. Valerian. *Am Fam Physician.* 2003; 67:1755-1758.

24   Abdelhameed AS, Ang S, Morris GA, *et al.* An analytical ultracentrifuge study on ternary mixtures of konjac glucomannan supplemented with sodium alginate and xanthan gum. *Carbohydrate Polymers.* 2010; 81: 141-148.

25   Harding SE, Smith IH, Lawson CJ, Gahler RJ, Wood S. Studies on macromolecular interactions in ternary mixtures of konjac glucomannan, xanthan gum and sodium alginate. *J. Carbpol.* 2010; 10:1016-1020.

26   Brand-Miller JC, Atkinson FS, Gahler RJ, *et al.* Effects of PGX®, a novel functional fibre, on acute and delayed postprandial glycaemia. *Eur J Clin Nutr.* 2010 Dec; 64(12):1488-93.

27   Jenkins AL, Kacinik V, Lyon MR, Wolever TMS. Reduction of postprandial glycemia by the novel viscous polysaccharide PGX® in a dose-dependent manner, independent of food form. *J Am Coll Nutr.* 2010; 29(2):92-98.

28   Vuksan V, Sievenpiper JL, Owen R, *et al.* Beneficial effects of viscous dietary fiber from Konjac-mannan in subjects with the insulin resistance syndrome: results of a controlled metabolic trial. *Diabetes Care.* 2000; 23:9-14.

29   Reimer RA, Pelletier X, Carabin IG, *et al.* Increased plasma PYY levels following supplementation with the functional fiber PolyGlycopleX in healthy adults. *Eur J Clin Nutr.* 2010 Oct; 64(10):1186-91.

30   Lyon MR, Reichert RG. The effect of a novel viscous polysaccharide along with lifestyle changes on short-term weight loss and associated risk factors in overweight and obese adults: an
observational retrospective clinical program analysis. *Altern Med Rev.* 2010 Apr; 15(1):68-75.

31   Freeman MP, Rapaport MH. Omega-3 fatty acids and depression: from cellular mechanisms
to clinical care. *J Clin Psychiatry.* 2011 Feb; 72(2):258-9.

32   Buydens-Branchey L, Branchey M, Hibbeln JR. Associations between increases in plasma n-3
polyunsaturated fatty acids following supplementation and decreases in anger and anxiety in
substance abusers. *Prog Neuropsychopharmacol Biol Psychiatry.* 2008; 32:568-575.

33   Kiecolt-Glasera JK, Beluryc MA, Andridged R, Malarkeya WB, Glasera R. Omega-3 supplementation lowers inflammation and anxiety in medical students: A randomized controlled
trial. *Brain Behavior Immunity.* Available online 19 July 2011doi:10.1016/j.bbi.2011.07.229.

34   Rudin DO. The major psychoses and neuroses as omega-3 essential fatty acid deficiency syndrome: substrate pellagra. *Biol Psychiatry.* 1981; 16:837-50.

35   Steptoe A, Butler N. Sports participation and emotional well-being in adolescents.

36   Moncrieff J, Cohen D. Do antidepressants cure or create abnormal brain states? *PLoS Med.*
2006 Jul; 3(7):e240.

37   Middleton H, Moncrieff J. 'They won't do any harm and might do some good': time to think
again on the use of antidepressants? *Br J Gen Pract.* 2011 Jan; 61(582):47-9.

38   Möller HJ. Is there evidence for negative effects of antidepressants on suicidality in depressive
patients? A systematic review. *Eur Arch Psychiatry Clin Neurosci.* 2006 Dec; 256(8):476-96.

39   Fournier JC, DeRubeis RJ, Hollon SD, Dimidjian S, Amsterdam JD, Shelton RC, Fawcett J.
Antidepressant Drug Effects and Depression Severity: A Patient-Level Meta-analysis. *JAMA.*
2010; 303(1):47-53.

40   Schwartz TL, Nihalani N, Jindal S, Virk S, Jones N. Psychiatric medication-induced obesity:
a review. *Obes Rev.* 2004;5(2):115-21.

41   Raeder MB, Bjelland I, Emil Vollset S, Steen VM. Obesity, dyslipidemia, and diabetes with
selective serotonin reuptake inhibitors: the Hordaland Health Study. *J Clin Psychiatry.* 2006;
67(12):1974.

42   Byerley WF, Judd LL, Reimherr FW, *et al.* 5-Hydroxytryptophan: a review of its antidepressant
efficacy and adverse effects. *J Clin Psychopharmacol.* 1987; 7:127-137.

43   Poldinger W, Calanchini B, Schwarz W. A functional-dimensional approach to depression:
serotonin deficiency as a target syndrome in a comparison of 5-hydroxytryptophan and fluvoxamine. *Psychopathology.* 1991; 24:53-81.

44   Baldessarini RJ. Neuropharmacology of S-adenosyl-L-methionine. *Am J Med.* 1987; 83(suppl
5A):95-103.

45   Nguyen M, Gregan A. S-adenosylmethionine and depression. *Aust Fam Physician.* 2002;
31:339-343.

46   Kagan BL, Sultzer DL, Rosenlicht N, *et al.* Oral S-adenosylmethionine in depression: a randomized, double-blind, placebo-controlled trial. *Am J Psychiatry.* 1990; 147:591-595.

47   Gilliland K, Bullock W. Caffeine: a potential drug of abuse. *Adv Alcohol Subst Abuse.* 1984;
3:53-73.

48   Greden J, Fontaine P, Lubetsky M, *et al.* Anxiety and depression associated with caffeinism among psychiatric inpatients. *Am J Psychiatry.* 1978; 135:963-966.

49   Neil JF, Himmelhoch JM, Mallinger AG, *et al.* Caffeinism complicating hypersomnic depressive episodes. *Compr Psychiatry.* 1978; 19: 377-385.

50   Charney D, Heninger G, Jatlow P. Increased anxiogenic effects of caffeine in panic disorders. *Arch Gen Psychiatry.* 1985; 42:233-243.

51   Bolton S, Null G. Caffeine, psychological effects, use and abuse. *Orthomol Psychiatry.* 1981; 10:202-211.

52   Kreitsch K. Prevalence, presenting symptoms, and psychological characteristics of individuals experiencing a diet-related mood disturbance. *Behav Ther.* 1985; 19:593-594.

53   Christensen L. Psychological distress and diet – effects of sucrose and caffeine. *J Appl Nutr.* 1988; 40:44-50.

54   Abdoua AM, Higashiguchia S, Horiea K, *et al.* Relaxation and immunity enhancement effects of Gamma-Aminobutyric acid (GABA) administration in humans. *BioFactors.* 2006; 26:201-208.

55   Coleman CI, Hebert JH, Reddy P. The effects of Panax ginseng on quality of life. *J Clin Pharm Ther.* 2003; 28:5-15.

56   Davydov M, Krikorian AD. *Eleutherococcus senticosus* (Rupr. & Maxim.) Maxim. (Araliaceae) as an adaptogen: a closer look. *J Ethnopharmacol.* 2000; 72:345-393.

57   Hallstrom C, Fulder S, Carruthers M. Effect of ginseng on the performance of nurses on night duty. *Comp Med East West.* 1982; 6:277-282.

58   Shevtsov VA, Zholus BI, Shervarly VI, *et al.* A randomized trial of two different doses of a SHR-5 *Rhodiola rosea* extract versus placebo and control of capacity for mental work. *Phytomedicine.* 2003; 10:95-105.

59   Darbinyan V, Kteyan A, Panossian A, *et al. Rhodiola rosea* in stress induced fatigue – a double blind cross-over study of a standardized extract SHR-5 with a repeated low-dose regimen on the mental performance of healthy physicians during night duty. *Phytomedicine.* 2000; 7:365-371.

60   Spasov AA, Wikman GK, Mandrikov VB, *et al.* A double-blind, placebo-controlled pilot study of the stimulating and adaptogenic effect of *Rhodiola rosea* SHR-5 extract on the fatigue of students caused by stress during an examination period with a repeated low-dose regimen. *Phytomedicine.* 2000; 7:85-89.

61   Olsson EM, von Schéele B, Panossian AG. A randomised, double-blind, placebo-controlled, parallel-group study of the standardised extract shr-5 of the roots of *Rhodiola rosea* in the treatment of subjects with stress-related fatigue. *Planta Med.* 2009 Feb; 75(2):105-12.

62   Auddy B, Hazra J, Mitra A, Abedon B, Ghosal S. A standardized *Withania somnifera* extract significantly reduces stress-related parameters in chronically stressed humans: A double-blind, randomized, placebo-controlled study. *JANA.* 2008; 11:50-6.

63   Akhondzadeh S, Kashani L, Fotouhi A, *et al.* Comparison of *Lavandula angustifolia Mill.* tincture and imipramine in the treatment of mild to moderate depression: a double-blind, randomized trial. *Prog Neuropsychopharmacol Biol Psychiatry.* 2003; 27:123-7.